What Do I Say?

What Do I Say?

Talking with Patients about Spirituality

Elizabeth Johnston Taylor

Foreword by Christina Puchalski, M.D.

TEMPLETON *T* FOUNDATION PRESS

Philadelphia and London

Templeton Foundation Press
300 Conshohocken State Road, Suite 670
West Conshohocken, PA 19428
www.templetonpress.org

Typeset and designed by Kachergis Book Design

*Templeton Foundation Press helps intellectual leaders and others learn about science research
on aspects of realities, invisible and intangible. Spiritual realities include unlimited love,
accelerating creativity, worship, and the benefits of purpose in persons and in the cosmos.*

978-1-59947-117-4 (paperback, with DVD)
978-1-59947-120-4 (paperback, without DVD)

LIBRARY OF CONGRESS CATALOGING-IN-PUBLICATION DATA
Taylor, Elizabeth Johnston.
    What do I say? : talking with patients about spirituality / by Elizabeth Johnston Taylor.
      p. ; cm.
    Includes bibliographical references.
    ISBN 978-1-59947-117-4 (pbk. : alk. paper) 1. Medical personnel and patient.
2. Interpersonal communication.   3. Communication in medicine.   4. Medicine—
Religious aspects.   5. Spiritual care (Medical care)   6. Spirituality—Health aspects.
7. Medical personnel—Religious life.   8. Patients—Religious life.   9. Spiritual healing.
I. Title.
    [DNLM: 1. Professional-Patient Relations.   2. Spirituality.   3. Communication.
4. Religion and Medicine. WM 61 T239w 2007]
    R727.3.T39 2007
    610.69′6—dc22
                                                                            2006035802

Printed in the United States of America

07   08   09   10   11   10   9   8   7   6   5   4   3   2   1

To my daughters
   Rilla Kathryn and Elissa Lynn
gracious gifts of God.

Thank you for teaching me as I learn how
to talk with you about spirituality.

Contents

Foreword

Spirituality is essential to healthcare. Why? Illness, life stress, and loss can trigger profound spiritual questions in people's lives that address the very core of one's humanity: who am I and why am I here on earth? These questions can provoke deep crisis in people and, if these questions are not addressed, people can become hopeless and full of despair. Viktor Frankl wrote that spirituality is the essence of each human being. He also found from his experiences during World War II that people can cope with suffering if that suffering has meaning. It is the meaning that people find in the midst of suffering, loss, and illness that provides opportunities for growth, love, and peace.

Physicians, nurses, and other healthcare professionals have a tremendous potential to impact the lives of patients by attending to patients' spiritual needs and issues. By being present to patients in the midst of those "why" questions, we can help people move from despair to hope and from isolation to love. Dr. Elizabeth Johnston Taylor helps guide healthcare professionals with the skills needed to console patients as they navigate through often lonely and hopeless situations in their lives.

Spirituality can be defined as that part of people that seeks ultimate meaning in life, especially in the midst of suffering. That expression can take many forms—God, church, nature, spiritual beliefs, and values. Spirituality is that part of one's life that gives one awe and an awareness of something greater than one's life alone. It helps all of us touch upon the mystery of life and of death. Spirituality, at its core, is relational. Thus, it underlies the very nature of who we are as people in community—communities at home, work, places of worship, and with friends. Healthcare is a community as well. And to become a compassionate system of care, it is essential that spirituality be at the foundation of that system. Healthcare was founded to serve others, to help them in the midst of their greatest needs. Yet, today's healthcare system is lacking compassion and lacking an emphasis on service and love.

People need skilled medical and technical care that comes from a framework of patient-centered medicine, where the patients' beliefs and values are as integral to their care as their physical and emotional symptoms. And, even if a cure is not possible, there can always be an opportunity for healing, which can best occur in the context of love and compassion for one another. Thus, as Dr. Taylor describes, in order to be a healer, every healthcare professional needs to reflect on his or her own woundedness and the need to heal. In this way, we form a bond with our patients in a community of people who seek meaning and purpose in the midst of life's difficulties. Out of our loving presence to those whom we serve, healing can come about for the healthcare professional and the patient.

Christina M. Puchalski, M.D., O.C.D.S.
Associate Professor of Medicine and Healthcare Sciences
Associate Professor of Health Leadership and Management
Director, The George Washington Institute for Spirituality and Health
The George Washington University

Acknowledgments

Thanks to the John Templeton Foundation, which generously funded the process of developing and testing this curriculum; and,

To the panel of spiritual care experts who graciously contributed ideas and materials for this curriculum: Wil Alexander, M.Th., Ph.D.; Jim Dyer, L.C.S.W.; Carla Gober, Ph.D., M.A., R.N.; Henry Lamberton, Psy.D., M.Div., all of Loma Linda University, Loma Linda, CA; and to Brenda Simonds, M.Div., ACPE supervisor, Arcadia Methodist Hospital, Arcadia, CA; and

To the reviewers who supportively provided feedback on the workbook: Betsy Barber, Psy.D., associate professor of spirituality and psychology, Talbot School of Theology, Biola University, La Mirada, CA; Harleah Buck, B.S.N., R.N., doctoral student, University of South Florida, Tampa, FL; K. C. Carrigg, Ed.D., R.N., associate professor, School of Nursing, Loma Linda University; Gail DeBoer, M.S., R.N., assistant professor, Samuel Merritt College, Oakland, CA; Ramona Perez Greek, Ph.D., R.N., assistant professor, School of Nursing, Loma Linda University; Nancy Haugen, Ph.D., R.N., professor and chairperson, Department of Nursing, Florida Hospital College of Health Sciences, Orlando; Marilyn Herrmann, Ed.D., R.N., dean, School of Nursing, Loma Linda University; Cathy Horinouchi, M.S., R.N., assistant professor, School of Nursing, Loma Linda University; Pejman Kataeri, D.O., resident, Pediatric Medicine, Loma Linda University Medical

Center; Terry Larsen, M.S.N., R.N., C.N.S., P.H.N., C.E.N., doctoral student, University of San Diego, San Diego; Iris Mamier, R.N., doctoral candidate, School of Nursing, Loma Linda University; Gail Rice, Ed.D., Ed.S., R.N., C.H.E.S., professor of allied health studies, Loma Linda University; Charlotte Schober, M.S.N., R.N., associate professor, Union College, Lincoln, NE; Wendy Stiver, B.S.N., M.A., R.N., O.C.N., oncology care coordinator, Arcadia Methodist Hospital, Arcadia, CA;

To Aaron Bacall, cartoonist, abacall@msn.com, for his playful and insightful visual reflections; and

To Laura Barrett, managing editor, Templeton Foundation Press, for her vision and careful guidance.

What Do I Say?

1 Let's Begin!

You've heard it:

"Why is this happening to me?"

"Am I dying? Am I going to be okay?"

"Why should I live? I'm just a burden to others."

"If I just pray harder, a miracle will happen."

"I did this to myself—I just can't forgive myself."

Whether patients are expressing a need to make sense of tragedy, find hope for the future, ascribe purpose and worth to living, trust religious beliefs, or relate to self and others with love, they are telling us about their inner spiritual needs. These needs are often deeply painful.

Such painful expressions of the human spirit often perplex and overwhelm the listener. This spiritual pain is often too hard to hear. Undoubtedly, when you have listened, you've heard patients—and even your friends and family—say things that left you wondering, "What do I say?"

This workbook will help you to answer this very question. In addition to providing you with suggestions for how to form healing verbal responses to expressions of spiritual pain, this workbook offers exercises for practicing and applying your newfound knowledge. Learning these communication skills are fundamental, but they will not be helpful unless you practice them. The adage "practice makes perfect" applies!

Why should I learn this skill?

The inner discomfort you have when patients express their spiritual pain may be motivating you to complete this workbook. There are, however, evidence-based reasons why health care professionals (HCPs) should learn this skill.

Emotional expression promotes spiritual healing.

Emotional expression is an avenue for accessing and expressing one's spirituality. "Opening up" and sharing deep emotions has been shown to contribute to physical as well as to emotional healing.[1] By helping patients express their innermost feelings and spirituality, health care professionals promote healing.

HCPs, furthermore, are in a unique position to help patients. Not only do they often meet patients during times of chaos and challenge, they meet patients as strangers. Strangers don't have the "baggage" that family and friends have. With HCPs, patients do not have a history of relating within established rules, so they often feel it is safer to share unspoken fears and secret feelings with health care professionals.

Spiritual health is related to physical and emotional health.

Hundreds of research studies have suggested a relationship between religiosity or spiritual health and physical health.[2] Although these studies vary significantly in quality and methodology, the evidence tentatively supports the longstanding theoretical models that link body, mind, and spirit. Science appears to verify Plato:

As you ought not to attempt to cure the eyes without the head, or the head without the body, so neither ought you to attempt to cure the body without the soul . . . for the part can never be well unless the whole is well. . . . And therefore, if the head and body are to be well, you must begin by curing the soul.[3]

Spiritual coping promotes adaptation to illness.

Patients frequently use spiritual coping strategies to manage their illness experience.[4] These coping strategies, like prayer, meditation, scripture reading, and clinging to comforting religious beliefs, are usually considered very important and meaningful to patients. While evidence suggests that use of positive religious coping is directly correlated with health outcomes, other evidence indicates that patients recognize that these coping strategies do not magically cure or substantially reduce symptoms. By facilitating patient use of healthful spiritual coping, clinicians promote adaptation.

Patients want their health care professionals to know about their spirituality.

Many patients appreciate having HCPs show concern for their spiritual health.[5] Patients with a serious or life-threatening condition, patients who are religious, and patients who perceive they have some relationship with the clinician are especially receptive to inquiries about their spiritual health. Although nurses and physicians are not viewed as primary spiritual caregivers and patients often do not want to be explicitly asked about their beliefs or invited to participate in intimate religious practices, most patients do want their health care professionals to know about their spirituality.

A nonempirical reason for learning to provide spiritually healing responses to patients is that, in addition to helping patients, we help ourselves. Psychotherapist John Sanford wrote that "by making a mature response in a difficult situation we become more mature . . . you are what you do."[6] As you complete this workbook, you may discover the journey is more about answering your own spiritual questions rather than those of patients.

About this workbook

This workbook is designed for HCPs—nurses, physicians, and allied health professionals, especially. Social workers, chaplains, clergy, and others who may get some training in counseling may also find this workbook beneficial. This curriculum is intended for those who provide care to primarily adults without mental illness. Although the content can be useful in some pediatric and mental health contexts, caring in such settings requires additional knowledge and skills that are not addressed here.

This workbook will require about ten hours to complete. Racing through the workbook, however, is not recommended. Allow yourself time to enjoy the process and to reflect on how you will integrate the knowledge and skills into your life. You may choose to complete one chapter a month, for example.

This book integrates knowledge from several disciplines, including psychology, psychiatry, pastoral counseling, nursing, chaplaincy, and spiritual direction. Although Western and Judeo-Christian experience typically influences the thinking on this topic, the workbook keeps the varied spiritual experiences of patients and HCPs in mind. Although institutionalized religion is an expression of human spirituality and an aid to spiritual formation, it is distinct from the broader concept of spirituality. Spirituality is universal, innate in all individuals. Kenneth Pargament, for example, defined spirituality as "a search for significance in ways related to the sacred."[7]

"God" language is used in this book. It is not intended to confine the reader to a prescribed Judeo-Christian orientation. Readers can substitute words and ideas that represent the transcendent for them, the sacred or holy (e.g., Spirit, Ultimate Other, Sacred Source, Higher Power). Patients, of course, often use the term God. The word "patient" is used in this workbook to denote any recipient of care, including family members.

Not only does a person's culture greatly influence how he or she experiences and expresses spirituality, culture also influences how patients talk about their spirituality with an HCP. A thorough description of how culture can affect conversations about spiritual matters is beyond the scope of this book. However, the following general principles for conversing with a patient from a culture other than your own should be remembered:

- Maintain an attitude—and, consequently, behaviors—of respect. This should begin the moment you meet a patient, when you use his or her proper name.

- Mirror patients' communication behaviors. Remain sensitive especially to the use of touch and eye contact, as their meaning varies between cultures. For example, Hispanics usually welcome handshakes and hugs, whereas many from Southeast Asia minimize touching.

- Follow a patient's lead on a topic. While some persons from Western, future-oriented cultures like to get to the point, others cultures may practice subtle and slow approaches to discussing concerns. Likewise, while some will want to talk openly about sensitive issues like dying, others may believe such topics are to be avoided.[8]

- The bigger the crisis, the less culture will affect clinician-patient interaction. For example, Asians who normally restrain strong emotions will likely want someone to pour out their soul to if they are in crisis.

This book addresses the question of how to form healing verbal responses to patients' expressions of spiritual pain. Although offering healing verbal responses is a fundamental skill for health care professionals, it is not the only approach for nurturing the spirit. Being silently present, reading inspirational materials, offering prayer, and encouraging journal writing or dream analysis are examples of other approaches. To learn about these and other spiritual care therapeutics, consult a text on spiritual care for HCPs.[9]

Assumptions

Many assumptions underlie the content of this workbook. They include:

1. Spirituality is an innate, universal dimension that integrates all humans.[10]

2. Healing is about promoting health, even if in only incremental and immeasurable amounts.

3. Healing involves attending to the health of the body, mind, and spirit. Because the body, mind, and spirit are interrelated, spiritual healing can affect physical and emotional health—and vice versa.

4. The goal of healing, ultimately, is to assist persons to experience existence more fully; to die living, rather than to live dying.[11]

5. Living fully requires self-awareness.[12] Self-awareness involves intellectual, emotional, and bodily awareness; these forms of self-awareness allow spiritual and God awareness—and a state of being at ease (instead of dis-ease). Self-awareness allows one to unblock distressing feelings and sort things out for oneself to surmount challenges.[13] Many recognize self-awareness and healing as a God-given grace.

6. "Whether he is called or not, the God will be present" (quote purportedly displayed in Carl Jung's office).[14]

7. The ability to heal reflects the degree of personal self-awareness and compassion experienced by the healer. Healers' spiritual awareness motivates them toward compassionate responses to patients.

8. Healers recognize healing results from "God's work *through* the relationship rather than from their own purely au-

tonomous efforts."[15] Consequently, healers carry no burden of responsibility for patients' healing.[16]

The goal of this workbook, therefore, is to teach HCPs to provide responses to patients that allow patients to become intellectually, emotionally, and physically aware of their spirituality so that they can experience life more fully. Figure 1.1 illustrates this framework and identifies where in this workbook you will learn about various approaches to increasing awareness.

EXERCISE 1.1

Think about a time when you were with a distressed patient and you found yourself asking, "What do I say?" Write the incident down here by writing word for word, as best as you can remember, what the patient said or did that prompted the question. Be sure to protect the anonymity of the patient by using a pseudonym.

FIGURE 1.1. Model for Supporting Patient Spiritual Health

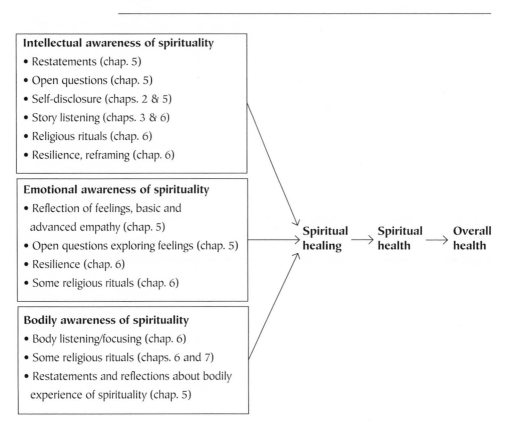

Intellectual awareness of spirituality
- Restatements (chap. 5)
- Open questions (chap. 5)
- Self-disclosure (chaps. 2 & 5)
- Story listening (chaps. 3 & 6)
- Religious rituals (chap. 6)
- Resilience, reframing (chap. 6)

Emotional awareness of spirituality
- Reflection of feelings, basic and advanced empathy (chap. 5)
- Open questions exploring feelings (chap. 5)
- Resilience (chap. 6)
- Some religious rituals (chap. 6)

Bodily awareness of spirituality
- Body listening/focusing (chap. 6)
- Some religious rituals (chaps. 6 and 7)
- Restatements and reflections about bodily experience of spirituality (chap. 5)

Spiritual healing → **Spiritual health** → **Overall health**

2 Preparing the Healer

Only *wounded* health care professionals can heal. This centuries-old idea has been argued by many, for example:

One's own hurt, one's sensitive openness to the patient, gives the measure of one's power to heal.[1]

Who can save a child from a burning house without taking the risk of being hurt by the flames? Who can listen to a story of loneliness and despair without taking the risk of experiencing similar pains in his own heart and even losing his precious peace of mind? In short: "Who can take away suffering without entering it?"[2]

Health care professionals (HCPs) cannot hear, never mind respond, to a patient's spiritual pain unless they hear and respond to their own pain. Thus, the purpose of this chapter is to help you recognize your own spiritual pains and appreciate that your pains parallel those of your patients. Valuing your woundedness is a necessary foundation for listening and responding to patients in ways that are healing.

What are my spiritual pains?

You may be thinking, "But I don't feel any spiritual pain!" Or, you may be overwhelmed by pains and be wondering how any of them could possibly help you to heal. The next two exercises are designed to help you become more aware of your spiritual pains.

EXERCISE 2.1

This exercise is an adaptation of one that Dr. Henry Lamberton uses with medical students at Loma Linda University. Check the answers that best reflect your innermost wants and how well these desires are satisfied. Circle the wants that you think most people would check.

What do I really want?	How strong is this want?			How satisfied am I that I have it?		
	1 Weak	2 Moderate	3 Very strong	1 Very unsatisfied	2 Moderately satisfied	3 Very satisfied
To be able to authentically love others			✓		✓	
✓ **To be loved by others**			✓		✓	
To be known		✓			✓	
✓ **To make a difference**			✓		✓	
✓ **To be safe (physically, emotionally, financially)**			✓		✓	
✓ **To be cherished by another**			✓			✓
✓ **To have meaning for living**			✓		✓	
✓ **To be respected**		✓				✓
To have serenity			✓			✓
✓ **To have power, influence**	✓					✓
Other _____						

How similar are your responses to those you assume others would give?

Consider what might be your most unsatisfied, or most pressing, innermost desire. This could be your primary spiritual theme or need. *future financial safety*

- How does it affect your interactions with others?

- How does it affect where you place your time and energy? *When alone, I worry*

- How would you relate to a person who has the same spiritual theme? *- Empathise - Elicit fears. - Listen*

EXERCISE 2.2

"Practicing soul inquiry" exposes the heart and allows one to become more spiritually self-aware.[3] Complete at least two of the following phrases; choose ones that unsettle you the most:

What is dying in me is _____

_____

This death is an intrusion in my life because_____

_____

What I want to scream about is _____

_____

My faith is challenged because_____

_____

I weep for _my saddness, feelings of fear, afeeling that I must earn money_

What I need to be unbound from is_____

_____

What paralyzes me, makes me indecisive is_ needing to do it right Fear that I am not good enough_

What embitters me is_____

_____

What I fear losing control of most is _____

_____

How do my spiritual pains affect my responses to patients?

Your spiritual pains or woundedness can affect your care of patients either positively or negatively. You can choose the outcome.

A negative outcome can occur when an HCP who has not reflected on his or her inner experience tries to address the spiritual pain of a patient. Such HCPs may be unaware of, afraid of, or misunderstand their deeper feelings, so they are unable to accurately identify and explore patients' spiritual pains. When patients realize an HCP does not understand them, they clam up, change the topic, give superficial responses to queries, or in other ways indicate disinterest in continuing to talk about their spirituality. This type of experience can increase patients' mistrust of health care providers.

Your woundedness, instead, can become a bridge or tool for healing communication. A healing response requires recognizing a patient's innermost feelings. Awareness of your own deeper feelings—your own spiritual themes and inevitable woundedness—is requisite to being able to hear another's. Thus, an HCP's life story, with its joys and wounds, becomes a source of information for interpreting a patient's story. For example, a nurse who is frustrated because she thinks she has not made a difference in the life of a "noncompliant" patient can begin to understand the experience of a parent whose "noncompliant" diabetic teen enters the emergency department with ketoacidosis. Or the clinician who can recognize the death and finality of every moment can be a healing companion for a dying patient.

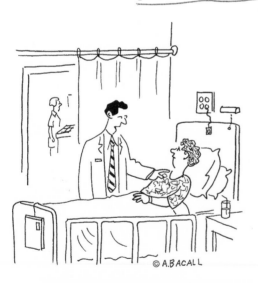

© A.BACALL

"Of course I'm listening to your expression of spiritual suffering. Don't you see me making eye contact, striking an open posture, leaning towards you and nodding empathetically?"

EXERCISE 2.3

Healers do not need to have had the same *experiences* as patients but, to be compassionate, they do need to recognize how they have shared similar *emotions*. Complete the empty boxes to learn how you and patients share deep emotions. Examples are provided.

Patient scenario	In what way can I relate? When have I *felt* this way?	Identify the shared deeper feeling/s
80 y/o SNF resident: "We had a fight a long time ago and he's never been close to me since then. He never comes to visit."	When a romantic interest broke up with me.	Rejection, abandonment, having love withheld by someone I really wanted it from.
56 y/o female with multiple sclerosis: "I'm so embarrassed to have to wear diapers now. I just can't predict when I'm going to pee in my pants. And the pain, when it comes, I just can't do anything to lessen it. I'm just losing control over my body!"	When I had the flu and nothing I did seemed to diminish its symptoms. Or, when I was pregnant and I just kept gaining weight and having my body do things I couldn't control, like stretch marks and sciatica. Or, when I was driving in the rain and my car went out of control.	Powerlessness. Unable to control something that is so very much a part of me and my identity, something that previously was very much under control.
Spinal cord–injured 22 y/o male: "I know I was going too fast on my bike but, my God! Why didn't he protect me? I'm so angry I could explode. My whole life is messed up."	Job loss (RIF) in school system. Why me? I had just bot my house — I had worked hard.	Abandonment. Faith shaken. Feeling alone. Fear of unknown. Fear won't get thru it. Fear things won't change
Family caregiver for adult cancer patient with pain: "I'm doing my best, but it doesn't seem to be good enough. I just don't know what to do. I can't stand to see him suffer."	Elaine - unsatiable request for attn. Nothing fills the hole.	- Helpless - Drained - Don't know what to do - Failure - Want to give up
48 y/o female hospice patient: "I know my husband will be okay after I leave. Sure, sad. So sad. But I just can't stand to think of my young kids without their mommy. [cries] Who's going to take care of them?"		

But if I'm always being wounded, won't I die?

By now, you may be wondering how can I be a wounded healer in the face of so much suffering? When I see so many human tragedies during my forty hours a week, week after week, how can I not weary of it? Being a health care provider to those who suffer can be overwhelming; their pains can suck us into a black hole of despair, and make us burn out!

You may have succumbed to an unhelpful attitude and way of coping that is prevalent. This perspective is described in an article published in a widely distributed nursing magazine: "Nurses must have compassion for their patients, but remain detached enough to do their job effectively. The very emotions that motivate people to become nurses are the same ones that must be suppressed . . . ," the article begins. At the end of the article, the author advocates, "Focusing on the specifics of that job will allow you to distance yourself and do what is best for the patient. Sometimes playing 'devil of mercy' is the ideal way to show you care."[4]

Before exploring how the HCP can remain wounded yet not die from the wounds, a clarification of the HCP's goal is in order. T. Hora argued:

The compassionate man says, "I love you because I understand you." The empathizing man says, "I know how you feel." The sympathizing man says, "I feel for you." Empathy and sympathy are . . . devoid of healing power. They have a temporary soothing effect, but they do not heal.[5]

Although some may squabble with this characterization of empathy, the goal for healers is, nevertheless, to understand the patient compassionately. Such compassion involves respecting patients' choices and ways of processing suffering; it does not involve controlling or manipulating the attitudes or solutions chosen by patients. Compassionate HCPs, therefore, are kept from burning out because they understand the limits of their responsibility and do not over-own patients' outcomes.

Suppressing, distancing, or desensitizing oneself from others' feelings involves walling off their painful feelings. Consequently, we lose the ability to hear and truly understand them. Although superficially helpful to the HCP, these responses are therapeutically ineffective for patients and, over the long term, contribute to losses for HCPs:

- Loss of information. Suppressing feelings means suppressing a source of information. So, when an HCP suppresses his or her feelings in response to seeing tragedy, he or she loses a resource that could otherwise help him or her to understand the patient's deepest feelings and needs.

- Loss of learning. The HCP likewise loses an opportunity to learn from the patient's experience. A healer is receptive to experiencing an internal change because of being with the patient. As a witness to a patient's spiritual suffering, the HCP—if engaged and open—can learn many spiritual lessons from the patient's experience. The HCP, for example, can learn about his or her vulnerability and impotence in the face of suffering. The HCP can also learn about his or her dysfunctional images of God (e.g., God as a rescuer or sugar daddy), about what is worth valuing, or about releasing the illusion of control.

- Loss of emotional control. When feelings are pushed into the HCP's unconsciousness, furthermore, they get pent up and explode later.[6] This explosion could be embarrassing and harmful to relationships the HCP wants to keep. Or they may not explode, but they may still influence interactions with patients. For example, unresolved ambivalence about religion can contribute to an HCP pressing antireligious feelings on a patient.[7]

- Loss of job satisfaction. Suppressed feelings and an inability to value the lessons a patient has to teach are often signs of professional burnout. Burnout has been described as "an erosion of the spirit. . . . It involves a loss of faith in the very enterprise of helping."[8]

Why do I disengage from patients' feelings?

Health care professionals typically choose their professions because they want to care, they want to help and heal others. And those who enter their professions most "on fire" to make a difference are at most risk for burnout. What causes a caring person to stop caring? Why do nice HCPs become numb to their clients? Why do they burn out?

Although many mechanisms contribute to burnout, there are some explanations that are essentially spiritual: Not being able to find meaning in one's work and feeling like one's effort does not make a difference leave a person vulnerable to burnout.[9] Grosch and Olsen[10] suggested that "masked narcissism" is at the root of burnout. That is, when one views work as a way of getting love (e.g., to gain self-esteem, gratification) rather than of giving it, burnout becomes possible. If this explanation offends you, remember that motives are always mixed. Alongside the narcissistic motives that are presumably in all who care for others are also motives reflecting genuine compassion.

To illustrate, when an HCP is overwhelmed by tragedy and feels he or she cannot make a difference to improve someone's life, the experience adds to the potential for burnout. When HCPs are unable to see how their work contributes to a meaningful outcome, their risk for burnout increases. When colleagues, supervisors, or patients fail to show their gratitude, give respect, or affirm self-worth, HCP burnout is more likely. These deep-seated threats expose HCPs' wounds. Unless HCPs reflect and learn from their experiences of woundedness, various cognitive defense mechanisms will be needed for "protection" against such threats. HCPs may, for example, mentally hide their sadness or anger, intellectualize the tragedies they see, or project their difficult feelings on others.

Reflect on the following questions:

In your life, how is the balance between giving care to others and receiving care from others?

I only give care   1 ---- ②--- 3 ----- 4 ----- 5   *I only receive care*

How often do you wish that patients would tell you that they appreciate the care you give them?   *They do .*

Very little or not at all   1 ----- 2 ----- 3 ----- 4 ----- 5   *Very much or a lot*

How often do you feel like what you've done at work has made a difference?

Very little or not at all   1 ----- 2 ----- 3 ----- 4 --- ⑤   *Very much or a lot*

How valuable do you think your work is?

Very little or not at all   1 ----- 2 ----- 3 ----- 4 --- ⑤   *Very much or a lot*

If you are discouraged about your work, you may want to jump to the last section of this chapter ("Tips for how to survive . . .," page 21) for some courage.

Assumptions that silence

Some HCPs hold assumptions that cause them to offer patients a silencing response, a response that shuts up patients.[11] These assumptions illustrate how our thinking can undermine our ability to heal.

- "I can't do anything about it." This also implies, "So why listen?"

- "If we talk about the tragedy, the patient will fall apart or be destroyed."

- "I will be destroyed if I hear about this tragedy."

- "Good things happen to good people." Implying, "so this one must have been bad." Or, put another way, people get what they deserve and deserve what they get.

- "This is too terrible to be true."

- "This shatters what I believe about the world—that is, that I'm safe, I have worth, there's meaning for everything."

- "If it happened to you, it could happen to me."

- "People should just be strong and get over it." Implication: suffer alone.

Larson described these issues as "interpersonal allergies."[12] Such allergies include the fears of: 1) our own death, 2) being hurt, 3) hurting others, and 4) being engulfed by others' problems. When we hold such assumptions or have such allergies, they affect our response to a patient. They cause us to change the subject, give pat answers, fake interest, and make other silencing responses, which are listed in Exercise 2.5.

EXERCISE 2.5

Check the box under the number that best represents your experience with patients.

How often do I . . .	1 nearly never	2 a little	3 some	4 quite a bit	5 nearly always
Change the subject, so that it is more comfortable to me?	✓				
Say something funny to lighten up a heavy conversation with a patient?	✓				
Minimize the patient's discomfort (e.g., "It couldn't be that bad")?	✓				
Fear what the patient is going to say?	✓				
Provide pat answers when a patient raises a distressing concern?		✓			

(Continued) **How often do I . . .**	**1** nearly never	**2** a little	**3** some	**4** quite a bit	**5** nearly always
Say something sarcastic to a patient?	✓				
Focus on tangential information that is unnecessary?		✓			
Try to fix patient problems by imposing my solution?		✓			
Avoid an uncomfortable topic?	✓				
Feel bored while listening to a patient talk?			✓		
Feel afraid that I won't be able to help?			✓		
Blame patients for their problems?		✓			
Feel numb towards a patient?	✓				
Impose positivity (e.g., "It's all going to work out")?	✓				
Wish the patient would just get over it?	✓				
Fake interest while listening to a patient?		✓			

Most of the questions above are adapted from an instrument developed by Baranowsky[13] to measure compassion fatigue. The higher your scores on these questions, the more likely you are experiencing compassion fatigue, a condition of being traumatized by witnessing or hearing about another's trauma.

What is a wounded healer like?

Effective helpers are like those who hold a candle in the darkness and then light another's candle with their flame.[14] These helpers do not make the other depend on their light. Neither do they give their candle away. Instead, the helper assists the other to brighten, to blossom, to flourish. So it is with the wounded healer.

Other features of the wounded healer are distinguished from traditional ways of thinking about helping in Table 2.1. These two paradigms are more like two ends of a continuum. Like neuroses (which can be managed but not cured), healers can over time move more fully into the wounded healer paradigm.

Table 2.1.   Wounded Healer vs. Conventional Paradigms Contrasted

Characteristics	Wounded healer paradigm	Conventional paradigm
Perspective	Helper	Fixer
	"I appreciate, understand, respect your pain, care about its affect on you, but cannot carry it for you."	"I feel your pain so much that some of it stays with me."
	"I'll walk beside you."	"I'll carry you."
Attitude of HCP during encounter	Curiosity, wonder Gratitude Reverence Sense of being on "holy ground"	Self-protective
		Needy of compliments, motivated by need to gain approval or by others' love and respect.
		Perceives failure if problem is not fixed (e.g., disease not cured).
	Relationship is symmetric; HCP is fellow traveler on road of life with patient.	Relationship is asymmetric; helper is more gifted, skilled, knowledgeable than patient.
Patient's experience	Able to trust even secrets and deepest pains.	Worried about overwhelming or incapacitating the helper.
	Finds load of carrying these burdens lightened by having named them.	Unable to fully trust helper, fearing he or she will back off.
	Feels companioned	Feels alone
Outcome for HCP	Blessed or better for the encounter	Emotionally weak, drained
	Can be physically tired, but internally joyful (even exhausted and sorrowful, yet at peace about the care provided).	Physically tired

Tips for how to survive in the clinical setting as a wounded healer

Several strategies, if implemented, can help the HCP to survive as a wounded healer instead of as a dying helper.

Find a way to address your own feelings.

If you can't talk openly with a counselor about your emotional responses at work, then write them in a journal or visit with a trusted friend.

Cultivate camaraderie with your colleagues.

Kill "staff infections." Being able to share successes and struggles at work offsets stress.

Allow for meaningful work experiences.

- Be curious. Learn more about what baffles. Appreciate the wonder of the body and the mystery of health.

- Introduce variety into your work

- Notice how clients *do* give back to you

- Notice and ask potential teachers (e.g., a challenge, flower, person's story): "What can I learn from you?"

- Say "that's a freebie" to all the unexpected gifts a day brings

- Have decompression time after work that allows reflection and making sense of what has happened to you

Recognize that you can affect change.

For example:

- You are only one, but $1 + 1 + 1 + 1 + \ldots$ means momentum for change.

- Be grateful for what you can do; don't ruminate about what you can't do.

- Make your goals realistic, achievable.

- Remember that you are not a savior.

- Pray the Serenity Prayer: "God, grant me the serenity to accept the things I cannot change, the courage to change the things I can, and the wisdom to know the difference."

Remember your human frailty and nurture yourself.

- Eat and drink nutritiously.

- Exercise.

- Get necessary sleep.

- Play and recreate.

- Find a healthy boundary for how much time you work. Live more simply if you decide to work less.

- Give yourself positive feedback, and don't expect it from others.

Support your own spirit.

Choose spiritual practices that increase your self-awareness, or greater awareness of the Divine immanent within you. This may involve practicing religious rituals that are meaningful.

Remember that the inner discomforts that we want to escape can actually be our teachers. Appropriate guilt can lead us to right wrongs. Loneliness can bring forth reconnections. Grief can remind us of the beauty of attachments.

EXERCISE 2.6

Develop a plan for nurturing your own spirit, for being at home in your heart. First, check the items that you currently incorporate in your life. Consider whether any of them need adaptation. Next, add any other activities that you sense would be important.

do ☑ For 5–10 minutes each day after work (e.g., while driving home), reflect on what you learned at work that day (turn off the car radio).

☐ Observe a sabbath every week. Refrain from work and busyness. Choose activities that allow rest and recreation.

☑ Visit a spiritual mentor every two to three months. Limit the conversation to matters of the heart.

☐ Read two spirit-nurturing books a year.

☑ Experience spiritual communion with others who share a similar spiritual experience twice a month (e.g., attending religious services).

✓ ☑ Spend the first waking moments of each day "centering" yourself (e.g., recommitting yourself to fulfilling what you believe is your primary purpose in life, acknowledging three things for which you are grateful).

add ☑ Go on a retreat of solitude once a year (e.g., at a spiritual retreat house, hiking in the wilderness).

☐ Play frivolously and seek healthful, nurturing pleasures for half a day every week.

☑ Do Yoga, Pilates, Tai Chi, or other body movement that helps you feel centered and appreciative of your body

add ☐ Express your innermost feelings through an artistic medium once a month.

add ☐ Keep a spiritual journal, writing your heart's responses to daily living, your dreams, and so forth.

_____

_____

_____

Post your plan on your calendar or in another spot where it will remind you of your commitment to be at home in your heart.

3 Listening
Beginning the Healing Response

It is impossible to provide a healing response to a patient when you have not first heard his or her spiritual pain. Not only is listening a prerequisite to a healing response, it *is* a healing response. L. A. Burton, a respected chaplain, shared: "To listen is to hear through all the noise and discover the quiet place where both pain and promise wait to speak their healing words . . . through being heard patients can experience their own sacredness and thus enter into a process of healing."[1]

A spiritual director explained how "we listen foremost in order to hear the other into speech. . . . It is also that weary, troubled, or hungry souls may discover a place that is safe enough for them to name the truth of their lives."[2]

A strong visual image that describes what listening can do may be helpful. Listening lances the psychic wound so that powerful, pent-up feelings can drain and healing can begin. Put another way, a listener is like the practice board tennis players (patients) use to perfect their strokes (identify sources of suffering and ways to adapt).[3]

Not only does listening initiate healing, it also contributes to illness prevention. When people are not heard, this lack of communication begets a sense of isolation, which begets "evil," which begets illness or the perpetration of evil behavior.[4] Such insight is reflected in the National Listening Association's description of listening as "the language of peace."[5]

Although listening typically involves making a few verbal responses to help patients feel heard, this chapter will focus specifically on the process of receiving and constructing meaning from what a patient says.

EXERCISE 3.1

The next time you are in a clinical setting, ask one or two patients what it is like to have a health care professional really listen. If you won't have an opportunity to speak with a patient, ask a close friend or answer these questions yourself. You can ask questions such as:

- How do you *know* when your HCP is listening? How can you tell?

- What does it *feel* like when your HCP seems to be really listening? What does it feel like when the HCP isn't listening? In addition to how it makes you feel emotionally, how does it make you feel physically?

Write the responses that really impressed you here:

_____

_____

_____

_____

_____

_____

_____

_____

_____

Dimensions of listening

There are various dimensions and depths with which you can listen and be present to a client.[6] These dimensions of listening include:

- Intellectual—the HCP is able to reiterate the intellectual or factual content of what the patient has said back in a way that the patient recognizes.

- Emotional—the HCP can identify and reflect back to the patient the deepest feelings or significance of what they have said.

- Physical—the HCP maintains an awareness of the nonverbal and postural messages sent from the patient's body (e.g., voice quality, posture, facial expressions, the look in his or her eyes), as well as the HCP's own body's physical responses to incoming messages (e.g., neck tension, flushed face, "knot" in the stomach). These messages then inform the HCP's responses. For example, a nurse feels exhausted and slumps her shoulders while listening to a patient talk about several losses. Such information can inform the nurse that the losses are tiring for the patient as well as for herself.

- Spiritual—the listener has an awareness of the holy in the relationship, a sense of divine presence, and consequently an openness to whatever transpires in the conversation. Stairs described it this way:

To listen for the spiritual dimension in every human experience and life circumstance requires listening with a definite spirit and intentionality. We are listening for more than what is consciously expressed. We are listening for the very voice, presence, or absence of God in the soul, the core of our lives where meaning is created.[7]

The expert spiritual caregiver will be able to listen using all four dimensions. Because of our humanness, however, it is unrealistic to expect ourselves to be able to always listen with all four dimensions.

EXERCISE 3.2

The next time you are able to observe health care professionals as they interact with patients, assess what dimensions of listening they use. Or consider what dimensions of listening you use with all those you encounter during the next day.

- What dimensions of listening seem most related to the speaker being heard?

- How many dimensions of listening can you incorporate in your intentional listening?

- Which dimensions of listening do you think are most difficult to incorporate? Why?

Jot your impressions down here:

_____

_____

_____

_____

_____

_____

_____

_____

_____

_____

_____

_____

_____

_____

_____

_____

_____

_____

What to listen for

Although you can think about what patients say to you faster than they can speak, you are receiving lots of multilayered information when you listen. Ultimately, you need to listen more for *feelings* than for thoughts, more for the *process* of speech than for its content. You may be asking, "But what should I be listening for?" The following list begins to answer this question. Amidst all that the patient is saying, try to tune in to the following:

What spiritual themes are present?

In the stories and information that patients offer, at least one spiritual theme is always beneath the facts.[8] Examples of spiritual themes include: the incessant need for attention, respect, love; betrayal or victimization; inadequacy or failure; struggle or supremacy against the odds; abandonment; and so forth. To illustrate, a middle-aged businessman who is in cardiac rehabilitation may boast throughout his stories about "beating the odds" (i.e., getting into a fraternity even though his grades were mediocre, getting a powerful position at work even though he didn't match the expected profile, remarrying after being heartbroken by an adulterous wife). This man's identity, his ideas about life's meaning, his values, and his response to illness are shaped by this underlying theme.

What are the patients' feelings?

Watch for indicators that can lead to deeper feelings.[9] These indicators include:

- Feeling words (e.g., "I'm heartbroken!" "I feel so alone").

- Emotion in the voice, as well as shifts in emotion (e.g., change in voice quality, strained or softened voice indicating a deeper level of feeling after a normal conversational voice).

- Emotion expressed in face or body (e.g., tears, look of fear in eyes, body changes toward fetal position).

- Protesting too much (e.g., with an underlying sense of desperateness to be convincing, "No! I am not angry . . . I'm really not, I just get upset once in a while, but I'm not an angry person and hardly ever get angry. No, I'm just fine—really!").

- Self-contradictions, which indicate inner conflict (e.g., "I just trust myself to God, he'll take care of me if I have faith. . . . I just keep praying and praying, fervently believing he's already healed me. . . . But I do still have this sickness . . .").

- Discussion of parental or other crucial need-satisfying relationships (e.g., adult patient talking about how "Dad was never there for me," or woman describing distance in her relationship with her husband or joy from being with her children).

Negative feelings are especially important to notice. These feelings are often hidden, yet they most need attention. Negative feelings get expressed when patients need to defend themselves and feel threatened by the topic, the situation—or you.

Where is the patient placing energy?

For example, what places in the conversation are accompanied by a quickened or slowed pace to dramatize what is being said, a stronger voice or an impassioned whisper, or some other vocal effect that inherently brings attention to what is important in the message? What is being said when the patient's eyes light up, tear up, or look away? Studying where the patient places energy informs the professional about what is meaningful to the patient and may require follow-up.

What metaphors does the patient use to describe experience?

Although metaphors may be the only way to express deeply inward spirituality, being on the lookout for a patient's use of overt metaphors can help the HCP identify a patient's inner feelings and spiritual concerns.[10] Many patients describe their spiritual development as "a journey." God may be described as "like a Father" (or a therapist or a best friend). Prayer may be a conversation, a dance, or "like talking to the ceiling." A bedridden patient may describe the spiritually challenging experience as "having cabin fever" or "like someone threw me into a pit and left me." Exploring the meaning of cabin fever and the feeling of being thrown away undoubtedly will lead the patient to increased self-understanding.

What sensory avenue dominates the patient's talk?

Persons tend to express themselves either visually (e.g., "I recognized . . ." or "I see . . ."), auditorily (e.g., "I could tell that . . ." or "I hear what you're saying . . ."), or kinesthetically (e.g., "I felt . . ." or "I get what you're saying"). Recognizing the dominate mode in each patient will help you to formulate responses using this mode, allowing you to connect better.[11]

Although there are several things to consider as you listen, keeping the following questions in mind as you listen can serve to summarize these considerations:

- What are the deepest feelings? What spiritual needs are being exposed?

- How is the patient describing his/her experience? How does this process inform me?

- Why is the patient telling me this, and why now? Why does the patient want me to know this?

Tips for how to listen

Spiritual care experts offer many specific suggestions about how to listen to an individual's spirituality.[12]

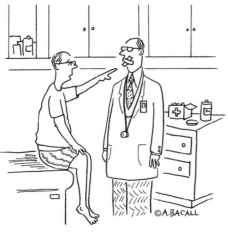

"Did you cut your lip while shaving or is that evidence you want to listen to me?"

Be curious! Want to hear the patient.

Patients will know if you really do not want to listen. Your listening will reflect such inner wishes. If you have only seventeen minutes to do your assessment, use those seventeen minutes to be fully present and listen (likewise, if you have only eighty seconds). You will be less efficient and less effective if you are a disengaged listener. If an HCP is in a hurry and acts as if he or she has only a few minutes to be with the patient, the problem will seem to take all day. In contrast, if you act as if you have all day, the problem will get fixed in a few minutes.[13]

Be authentic.

That is, don't wear a mask or build a façade. It hurts relationship building.[14] So, if you feel angry toward the patient, don't force a smile. If you want to cry and you know the tears are not about your own issues, let the tears come. Avoid flattery and other pretentiousness. Be genuine. Be you!

View the patient as a fellow human on a journey called life.

"Democratize the encounter"[15] and remember that you are not a savior. Rather, you are a fellow traveler.

Trust the patient.

Believe in the patient's inner resources and abilities for healing. Healers can't fix patients' spiritual suffering, but they can help patients access these assets.

Let the patient set the rules for the conversation.

When a patient's threshold for spiritual pain is exceeded, the patient will throw out an invitation to listen to it to someone—often, an HCP. The patient will wait to see if the HCP picks up on the invitation. Follow patients' cues about when to explore their spiritual experience more deeply with them.

Offer the patient safety as you listen.

Assure the patient you want to hear and be there (e.g., ask, "What are you thinking?"), and that you will not give up or leave him or her if you disagree. Avoid being judgmental, punitive, critical, or dogmatic. Avoid making false promises or giving false assurances.[16] Consider how we often show our conditional regard—"You don't think that . . . , do you?" or "Let's talk later"—when you do not have any specifics plans for doing so.

Do not interrupt.

When we finish another's sentence or cut in to change the flow of the conversation, we show impatience or discomfort. Interrupting is often a way to avoid or defend ourselves against something that is unpleasant.[17] A patient who describes religious beliefs with which you don't agree can easily push your interrupt button! Patients often describe their spiritual suffering through the telling of a story. For example, a woman who discusses going to the grocery store and becoming too tired to finish the shopping may be talking about her fear of losing independence and purposefulness. Instead of being inpatient with such trivial-seeming stories, allow the story to unfold.

Keep your story to yourself.

As a healer, your relationship with a patient is for therapeutic, not social, purposes. Do not interject your counter-story, boast, or make personal references. For example, "Yes, I know, I had that same experience when . . ." See chapter five of this workbook for guidelines on self-disclosure.

Maintain neutrality as you listen.

Even as you assure patients that you are there *for* them, maintain neutrality. For example, avoid exclamations of surprise or showing too much concern. Avoid approval or indifference. Instead, when you provide a neutral response, the patient won't know what you personally think is acceptable. For example, respond with "I'm guessing you feel elated about that" rather than "I'm so glad you did that!" A neutral response will help the patient to look within.[18]

Allow silence to do its work.

A patient's silence can mean different things. He or she may be thinking hard and choosing what to say next. This may indicate that he or she is struggling with something that is hard to put into words (often the case with spiritual matters). The patient may also be recovering from the exhaustion of emotional expression. Respect such silences; usually it is best to allow the patient to take the lead in restarting the conversation. It may be helpful, however, sometimes to let silence do its work and then follow it up with a gently spoken therapeutic response, such as, "You became very quiet after you asked 'Why?'" or "I'm wondering what the quietness means." You may even allow the patient time alone to reflect while you step out of the room. To assure the patient you are not abandoning him or her, however, you might say something like: "Our conversation has dealt with a very deep pain; I'm sensing that it might be best if I leave to allow you some time to reflect on it alone. I'll be back [state when] if that's okay with you." Allowing silence communicates to the patient that you will not run away or change the subject to a less uncomfortable topic if he or she stops talking. For some Native Americans, Arabs, and Europeans, your silence may be interpreted as a sign of respect and concern for privacy, or as agreement. When a patient's silence, however, means that he or she is waiting for information, reassurance, or interpretation from you, respond accordingly.[19]

Avoid worrying about what to say after the patient has finished talking.

Also, avoid premature interpretation and advice.[20] Many caregivers find comfort and confidence believing a divine Presence or Spirit will guide their response. Letting this "third party" do its job and practicing the techniques presented in this workbook will eradicate this obstacle to listening.

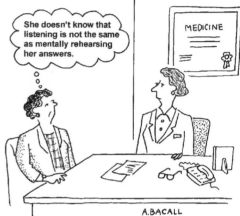

She doesn't know that listening is not the same as mentally rehearsing her answers.

MEDICINE

A.BACALL

Use body language to convey your interest in listening.

That is, maintain comfortable eye contact and a socially acceptable proximity. Of course, this varies among cultures. Euro-American counselors are taught to lean slightly forward, if possible, and face the patient from a 90–180 degree angle.[21] While Euro-Americans often interpret a lack of eye contact as reflective of dishonesty or discomfort, some Native Americans, Asians, and Muslims view prolonged eye contact as rude or invasive. Follow the patient's cues to determine appropriate body language. Keep your arms uncrossed, your feet and fingers still. If your body is conveying discomfort while you are talking with a patient about his or her spirituality, then you are feeling discomfort—and your patient will then mirror this discomfort. If necessary, take a deep breath and calm yourself before and during such uneasy conversation. And, of course, do not write in or read the patient's chart while listening!

Spend at least half to three-quarters of your time listening.[22]

A psychiatric adage is: "Listen to the story; therein lies the diagnosis."[23]

Use questions only when necessary.

Robert Carkhuff, a psychologist famous for studying empathic communication, taught that a therapeutic listener should not ask more than two questions in a row.[24] Questions often function to fill in conversation when the professional does not know what to say next. Avoid informational questions when listening to spiritual concerns; such questioning often leads to tangential material and consumes an HCP's precious time. Asking too many questions can also be a way to dominate a conversation; it takes initiative away from the patient.

Take comfort in the three strikes rule.

People typically give a listener three chances to hear them.[25] If they are not heard by the third try, they give up. If you fail to hear a patient's spiritual suffering, he or she will likely try again to tell you about it.

Overwhelmed? Now that you have read this list of listening techniques, you may be worried that it will be too hard to integrate them in your practice. Although using these techniques will greatly increase your effectiveness with a patient, do not worry about applying every technique offered here. Being anxious will decrease your ability to become aware of a patient's feelings and your response to them. Be comforted in knowing that a genuine sense of compassion for your patient will prevail over any "mistakes." Such compassion creates a healing environment.

EXERCISE 3.3

Quickly review the last section, "Tips for how to listen." Then choose the one suggestion that you think you most need to follow. Write how you intend to focus on this during your next listening encounter.

EXERCISE 3.4: INNER QUESTIONS FOR REFLECTION

Consider the following questions that Clinical Pastoral Education Supervisor Brenda Simonds gives to chaplain interns:

- Do I prefer speaking to listening? Do I resent not being the center of attention? Am I focused on how to respond when the patient is talking?

- Am I able to listen to radically different views (of life, God, values, beliefs) without being threatened? Do I feel compelled to defend or explain God?

- Am I able to differentiate between what a person says on the surface and his or her underlying meaning and/or concern? Can I listen for the music behind the words?

- Does how a person looks control my perception of what kind of person the speaker is or may become? Am I able to overcome personal differences to imagine myself in another's shoes?

- Do I shy away from hearing another person's problems, feelings (especially negative emotions)? Am I afraid of emotions—mine or others'?

- Do I find it difficult to admit my own limits and insecurities? Do I become defensive or angry when I feel helpless or inadequate?

- Am I genuinely interested in the lives of other people, curious about their experiences? Am I bored by or condescending to children, older adults, or people with mental illness?

- Do I have a greater need to be needed, loved, respected so that I do not have the capacity to care about and respect others?

- Is it possible for me to love a patient's soul without loving everything about him or her? Am I able to discern the brokenness behind the dysfunction?

EXERCISE 3.5

Consider the following interaction between a patient (PT) with chronic obstructive pulmonary disease (COPD) and a clinician (RN):

RN1: Well, you're about to be discharged. Do you have anyone to help you at home?

PT1: I live alone. My kids live in town, but they're too busy to help. The neighbors are new and I don't feel comfortable asking them. There's one guy at the church I used to go to that has helped me in the past, but since I don't attend anymore, I don't know if I should prevail upon him, you know what I mean?

RN2: Yeah, I know what you mean. It's kind of awkward. So why don't you go to church anymore?

PT2: Aw [looks away briefly, seems a bit nervous], I just haven't been for awhile.

RN3: So, how long has it been?

PT3: About a year.

RN4: Have you talked with anyone at the church recently to see if they could help you now?

PT4: [shrugs nonchalantly] Oh, they're happy to see me come.

RN5: Which one did you go to?

PT5: All Saints across town.

RN6: Oh. It's too bad, because you know they are now coming out with research that shows maybe going to church is related to being healthy.

PT6: Hmmm. Could be. So what do we need to do to get me out of here?

RN7: Please try to call someone at your church, because I know it is important to you. And a lot of our patients say that their religion comforts them at times like this.

PT7: [looks at floor, speaks unconvincingly] Okay. I'll think about it.

RN8: [cheerfully] I'll go get your discharge papers now. I'll be back in a minute.

Questions:

1. Circle at least two places in this verbatim where the patient indicates he does not feel heard.

2. What do you think the patient felt when the RN stated, "I know what you mean"?

_____

_____

_____

3. How similar are your listening skills to those of this nurse?

Not at all like this   1 ----- 2 ----- 3 ----- 4 ----- 5   *Very much like this*

Find an analysis in "Answers for Exercises," page 129.

4 Making Sense of What You Hear

As you listen to patients, you will hear overt and covert expressions of their spirit. But what do they sound like? How do you make sense of it? This chapter will train your ear for detecting and understanding the spiritual needs embedded in patients' conversations.

What are spiritual needs?

Several scholars have identified various categories of spiritual need.[1] Clinebell proposed four fundamental spiritual needs, which people have whether they are aware of them or not:

the need for a meaningful philosophy of life and a challenging object of self-investment, the need for a sense of the numinous and transcendent, the need for a deep experience of trustful relatedness to God, other people, and nature; and the need to fulfill the "image of God" within oneself by developing one's truest humanity through creativity, awareness, and inward freedom.[2]

In simpler language, humans all need:

1. meaning and purpose
2. to transcend self
3. healthy relationships
4. to be true to self

What does spirituality look and sound like?

Given that spirituality is an integral and integrating force within humans, it is natural that expressions of spiritual need and distress are embedded in "everyday" conversation and behavior. The stories patients tell, the ways they relate to their communities, their rituals, and so forth, all express the inner spiritual experience at some level.[3] Yet, because spirituality is experienced deeply and inwardly, it is often spoken of without awareness or expressed using metaphors and other figures of speech. Thus, expressions that hint at one's spirituality are vast and varied; for example:

- "I want to help others, so I'm going to that charity fundraiser" [purpose].

- "Everything happens for a reason" [meaning].

- "My kids are my life" [purpose, relationships with others].

- "I want to protect my family from seeing me suffer" [relationship].

- "I love looking at the stars at night; they remind me of my place in the universe" [awe, transcendence, meaning, relationship with nature].

- "My job is so unimportant, sometimes I wonder why I do it" [purpose].

- "I think God's trying to tell me something" [relationship, meaning].

- "I'm afraid of going to sleep, afraid I might never wake up" [authentic self, relationship with nature].

- "I don't know what to believe anymore" [meaning, relationship].

- "It's all in God's hands" [relationship, self-transcendence].

- "It's a celestial crapshoot" [meaning].

- Tears, anger, depression, withdrawal, avoidance of others [meaning, self-transcendence, relationship, authentic self].

- Smiling, peaceful demeanor [authentic, true self].

And so forth!

EXERCISE 4.1

Identify the spiritual need(s) expressed in the following statements. For example: A skilled nursing facility (SNF) resident as he is undressed by the nurse for a shower states: "I feel like such a baby having to be helped." His spiritual needs could include feeling worthless, helpless, vulnerable, dependent—indicators that he may need to connect in a healthy way with others (be loved, respected) or to become more aware and accepting of who he is. Or, to use Clinebell's language, he needs purpose, healthful relationships with others, and to appreciate his true (albeit physically dependent) self.

1. In the emergency room, the father of a twenty-one-year-old who has committed suicide: "I was always taught that taking your life was a sin. But now I can't see it that way. How could God not have mercy on my poor son?"

_____

_____

2. Spinal cord–injured patient in a rehabilitation unit: [with agony] "Why live? What do I have to offer now that I'm a quad?"

_____

_____

3. Cancer survivor who has just learned that a recent biopsy is negative: "Oh! I'm so relieved, so happy . . . so incredibly happy! Now I'm going to go and live my second life differently."

_____

_____

Answers are found in "Answers for Exercises," page 130.

Although you have not yet read the chapters about responding to patients' expressions of spiritual need, use the information you have just gained and circle which responses are best:

1. SNF resident: "I feel like such a baby having to be helped."

   A. *"Having to be bathed, I'm guessing, is humiliating."*

   B. *"Oh, so do you want me to shampoo your hair today?"*

2. In the emergency room, the father of a twenty-one-year-old who has committed suicide: "I was always taught that taking your life was a sin. But I know I can't see it that way. How could God not have mercy on my poor son?"

   A. *"Don't worry. Just commit it all to God."*

   B. *"Sounds like you're rethinking how you believe."*

3. Spinal cord–injured patient in a rehabilitation unit: [with agony] "Why live? What do I have to offer now that I'm a quad?"

   A. *"God wouldn't have let this happen if there weren't a purpose in it."*

   B. *"Seems you're distraught thinking that there may no longer be a reason for you to live."*

4. Cancer survivor who has just learned that a recent biopsy is negative: "Oh! I'm so relieved, so happy . . . so incredibly happy! Now I'm going to go and live my second life differently."

   A. *"I'm thrilled for you, too! What are you going to be with your new lease on life?"*

   B. *"Okay. Now don't forget your follow-up appointments."*

Answers are found in "Answers for Exercises," page 131.

Tips for making sense of what you hear

The following observations offered by spiritual care experts[4] provide guidance for gaining perspective about what patients say:

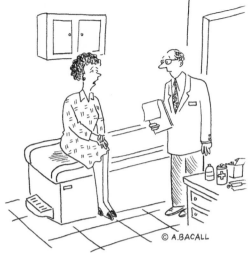

"You're not listening to what you're hearing."

Remember that what patients say to you at first reflects not how well you asked a good question, but how safe and respected the patient feels with you.[5]

At first, patients may describe their spiritual responses to illness using seemingly superficial idioms, such as, "The Lord has blessed me, I can't complain," "Allah is great!" or "Jesus is the answer." Such idioms can become springboards for exploration. For example, you can follow up with open questions or other micro-skills (see chapter five), such as: "How has the Lord blessed you?" "How do you experience Allah's greatness?" or "What answer does Jesus give you?" Or, when a patient resorts to "It's all in God's hands," you can encourage him or her to explore further by asking, "How safe is that?"

Consider what sorts of incongruities exist.[6]

Are there any incongruities between *a*ffect, *b*ehavior, and *c*ommunication (ABCs) shown by the patient? For example, is he saying, "I'm fine," while gritting his teeth? Also, does what the patient says about himself match what he wants to be? Does what he says match what he does? Do the patient's perceptions of self match your perceptions of him or her? Any incongruities you might observe suggest areas the patient may benefit from exploring, with you or with an expert. For example, "I noticed you gritting your teeth while you said that you were fine," or "You mentioned that God is in control and that you wish you could control how long you live. How is this for you?"

Consider the level of abstraction or concreteness of what the patient is saying.[7]

Patients who talk abstractly or conceptually are likely distancing themselves from thoughts and feelings they fear. For example, a patient who is avoiding recognition of feeling angry at God may say "God is love" and disengage from further probes that attempt to understand this abstract phrase. In contrast, when a patient uses concrete speech too much, it can indicate an anxiety about considering the more abstract meanings or implications of a belief. For example, the patient who describes dietary or other religious prescriptions in detail but is unable to explain the significance of these practices may be blocking it for a reason such as fear of divine condemnation. Healthy spirituality is illustrated by talk that straddles between the extremes of abstractness and concreteness.

Consider how defensive or threatened the patient is by talk about spirituality.[8]

People often show their anxiety about talking about spiritual matters by:

- Changing the subject (e.g., "Me feel angry? Naw, but it reminds me of someone who . . .").

- Talking superficially or about less important topics (e.g., "Oh, I just know it will all work out somehow").

- Making the professional do most of the talking (e.g., giving minimal answers that make the professional ask lots of questions or fill in the silences with talk, or by getting the professional to talk about him- or herself).

- Becoming competitive (e.g., patient starts quoting scripture or provides scriptural facts to show his or her knowledge).

- Intellectualizing feelings (e.g., "I know God loves me, but I can't feel it").

Such defensiveness is best countered by being present to patients as a sojourner in life, a fellow human dependent on God.[9]

Defensiveness may also be minimized by modeling comfort with talking about spirituality and by responding to the feelings and meanings of what the patient says (see chapter five for techniques). You may need to change the subject to a less threatening topic or recommend a referral to a spiritual care expert.

Keep in mind that crises expose the gaps in a patient's spiritual development.

For example, a man who during his childhood watched his favorite cousin drown and could not resolve how a loving God could allow it may become acutely aware of this unresolved spiritual issue when he is faced later in life with another tragedy. Healers allow patients to explore these gaps and grow through them.

Individuals develop spiritually, just as they do physically, cognitively, and ethically. Spiritual development involves learning about beliefs and practices concretely as a child, then abstractly as cognitive development allows. It involves learning from parents, then differentiating from these spiritual beliefs and practices as one enters the teenage years and young adulthood, and creating a satisfying personal belief system as one becomes an adult. Adult spiritual development often involves phases of re-searching for satisfying beliefs and meaningful practices.[10]

Remember that religion offers a lens for interpreting life.

When a person talks about religion, he or she is talking about his or her world.[11] For example, a patient who describes her faithful service to her church is not only telling you what she's proud of, but also about her values of commitment and perseverance, about something that provided structure and rhythm to her week, about what gave her life meaning and purpose, about what was worthy of her worship and what brought her respect, and so forth. Not only does religious talk portray a view of life, it also can reflect underlying emotional problems.[12] For example, an extremely pious patient actually may inwardly doubt her worth. Someone who is preoccupied with never "sinning" may be desperate for love and acceptance. Someone who tries hard to have an ecstatic religious experience may be trying to feel feelings that were suppressed during childhood. Someone who blames everything on an evil force or accepts that holy scripture has all the answers to all of life's problems may be showing his of her fear about taking responsibility or making tough decisions.

When patients share meaningful stories, legends, or passages from their holy scripture, they are telling you about themselves.

"Tell me what you find in the Bible, and I will tell you what you are."[13] How patients use and interpret their religion's scripture can be a diagnostic tool that informs HCPs about a patient's personality and beliefs. To illustrate, Sammy, a cancer patient, retells the story of Job:

Job's friends try to explain to him why God allows his tragedy to happen. Job doesn't find it helpful and feels like cursing God, but uses all his inner power to resist. He chooses to remain faithful. And in the end God restores his health, his family, and his fortune. Now isn't that a great story?

Sammy feels connected with Job. They share suffering and tragedy. Quite possibly, Sammy feels that his friends (e.g., his minister, family, colleagues) are like Job's. Sammy may be projecting his experience of spiritual isolation and his intellectualization of faith on Job. Likewise, Sammy appears to be taking comfort from the outcome Job had, and is probably hoping that his tragedy will end in earthly blessings as well.

Consider how helpful patients' spiritual beliefs and practices are.

Spiritual beliefs are helpful for patients to the degree that they foster personal emotional health, support positive relationships with others, and promote a hopeful involvement in the world.[14] "Life-enhancing religion [or spiritual beliefs] enables a person to confront rather than evade his existential anxiety. . . . Anxiety is the teacher who searches one's life thoroughly and roots out the trivial."[15] If unhelpful or dis-integrating religiosity is observed (see Table 4.1), a referral to a spiritual care specialist is recommended so that helpful spiritual coping skills can be enhanced. In the

Table 4.1. Unhelpful or Dis-integrating Religiosity[16]

Categories of unhelpful religiosity	Descriptions	Examples
Undifferentiated or one-sided religiosity	When persons pursue a narrow aspect of their religion, which keeps them from using a variety of religious coping strategies.	Focusing only on happiness-inducing beliefs and practices of a religion, to the exclusion of challenging or discomforting aspects (when confronted with suffering, will have difficulty finding helpful religious coping skills).
		Passively coping by leaving problems to "God's will" (may be unable to involve themselves collaboratively with God or HCPs while making health care decisions).
Fragmented religiosity	When persons live in a way that is disconnected from what is sacred in life; behavior is incongruent with spiritual beliefs.	Attending religious services on high holy days out of a sense of tradition, but failing to integrate the religious values espoused at services at home or work (when faced with suffering, such persons will have no meaningful beliefs or practices from which to find comfort).
Inflexible, rigid religiosity	Prevents persons from using various religious coping strategies and from considering various religious perspectives to interpret stressful circumstances.	Believing there are only certain correct ways to pray (may have difficulty praying when illness prevents the patient's usual approach toward God).
		Believing that "only one religion will get you to heaven" (may have difficulty when illness undermines a doctrine of that religion).
Insecure attachment to God	An anxious or unsure sense of connection with Higher Power, or what is sacred.	Dominating spiritual leader or spiritual community will make a person feel distant and alienated from what otherwise could be a strong source of support and comfort during stressful events.
		Feeling God or their parish has abandoned them.

meantime, remember that it would be cruel to unravel patients' unhealthy religiosity when it may be their only source of comfort. Use the micro-skills in chapter five to begin exploring their spirituality. For example, say, "Tell me more about what makes God feel so far away now."

These tips will help you make sense of what a patient is saying to you about his or her spirituality. This chapter posits that patient spirituality will naturally be reflected in varied topics of conversation. Therefore, there is little need for you to worry about what questions to ask patients to get them to talk about their spirituality. The techniques presented in the following two chapters will provide approaches to knowing what to say, including what to ask. For tips about initiating conversations about spirituality with patients, see chapter seven, FAQs 3 and 15. For questions to include in a spiritual assessment, consult chapter seven, FAQ 16.

EXERCISE 4.3

Analyze the following conversation excerpt between a health care professional (HCP) and a seventy-one-year-old patient (PT) receiving hospice care at home.

HCP1: How's your pain today?

PT1: I'm just praying and hoping that it'll go away.

HCP2: [assesses physical pain, discusses increasing dosage, encourages patients to take rescue doses]

PT2: Well, I'd just as soon suffer now than when I die. I'd just as soon go up there than down there [to hell].

HCP3: Tell me more about your beliefs about suffering, about living with pain.

PT3: I believe in being penalized for sins. I'm suffering now for sins I committed.

HCP4: You're thinking that your pain is a consequence of your past sins.

PT4: I dunno, maybe. [averts eye contact] You know, it's hard to say. There must be a reason I got it. It'd be easy if I knew why!

HCP5: You mentioned when I first came that you were praying about your pain. How do you relate to God when you're in such pain?

PT5: If I can concentrate, it takes my mind off the pain.

HCP6: Prayer is a distraction from hurting—when you can concentrate.

PT6: Yeah, I think it does, for a while anyways. It all depends on the man upstairs. If he wants me to have pain, I'm going to have it. And if I can't concentrate, then those prayers don't get answered.

HCP7: What do you think the man upstairs wants from you?

PT7: If I've suffered enough, he'll take you to heaven.

HCP8: Let me see if I'm understanding you. Your sense is that your pain is a result of your sin, and yet it also interferes with your praying or trying to reconnect with God.

PT8: Hmm. Hadn't thought of it that way, but guess you're right. Gotta think about that more.

HCP9: [after long pause] Let me know if you need a sounding board or a place to journal—how I can help you in your thinking.

Questions to prompt analysis:

1. How safe does the PT appear to feel with the HCP?

   Very unsafe   1 ----- 2 ----- 3   *Very safe*

2. How abstractly does the PT talk about his spirituality?

   Very concretely   1 ----- 2 ----- 3   *Very abstractly*

3. How defensive is the PT of his spiritual beliefs?

   Very defensive   1 ----- 2 ----- 3   *Not very defensive*

4. List two superficial religious idioms used by the PT.

   _____

   _____

5. Identify one incongruity evident in what the PT expresses.

_____

6. How does the PT use his religion? Describe how his religion is helpful or unhelpful.

_____
_____
_____

7. How helpful is the HCP?

Very unhelpful   1 ----- 2 ----- 3   *Very helpful*

See commentary in "Answers for Exercises," page 131.

5 Verbal Responses to Spiritual Pain

Micro-skills

This chapter presents the most fundamental "micro-skills" necessary for forming a healing verbal response to patients who express spiritual distress. Remember, however, that a verbal response may not be the best response to spiritual pain. It may be more helpful to remain wordlessly present, to give a knowing look or encouraging nod, or to cry and squeeze a hand. At some point, though, you will most likely sense that words are needed to foster healing.

The skills introduced in depth here are basic "helping," "attending," or "empathic listening" skills discussed in textbooks for beginning lay or professional counselors.[1] These skills can easily be used to help those in spiritual as well as in emotional distress. The somewhat linear process of helping is usually described as occurring in three stages: 1) facilitating exploration, 2) insight or understanding, and 3) action.

Given the limited time and expertise of most HCPs, an appropriate expectation is exploration when a patient expresses spiritual distress. In the process of exploration, some HCPs may foster insight and stimulate action. Although numerous basic helping skills exist, the skills most useful for exploration will be presented here: restatement, open questioning, reflecting feelings, and advanced empathy. Because patients often ask HCPs about their spiritual beliefs, self-disclosure will also be discussed. The first micro-skill introduced in this chapter, however, is one that is requisite to any healing response: rapport.

Micro-skills: Goals and guidelines

EXERCISE 5.1

Before continuing, write down what you think might be an acceptable verbal response for the following scenarios:

- Mother whose eleven-year-old daughter has just been diagnosed with Type I diabetes mellitus says: "Why do bad things happen to innocent children?"

_____

_____

- Woman with stage IV breast cancer says: "I've prayed so hard to be healed. . . . Maybe I'm praying in the wrong way."

_____

_____

- Eighty-seven-year-old home-care patient says: "I've just had so many friends and family die in the last few months. I don't know how much I can stand. I keep thinking maybe God is trying to teach me something, but I don't know what."

_____

_____

Goals

We cannot solve others' spiritual problems or even push them to solve their own. "The only real answer to human problems lies in each person's capacity to sort things out for himself [or herself]."[2] To sort things out, a person needs some self-awareness. People have varying degrees of awareness about how they think and feel about themselves. Helping skills can allow people to gain greater awareness of their thoughts, feelings, and the meanings of these feelings. Helping skills, therefore, help people to hear and understand themselves. An essential element of healing is the "working through" of distressing feelings.[3] When feelings are "blocked," healing is blocked. The following basic helping skills can be used to help patients unblock and work through their spiritual pain.

Solving others' spiritual problems, correcting or eliminating their spiritual suffering, and converting patients to your way of believing are inappropriate and unrealistic goals. Not only are these unethical approaches to caring, but they reflect what may be an unhelpful view of spiritual "problems." Spiritual problems are not things to solve, but opportunities for finding God (however God is experienced).[4] The goal of listening and responding to patients' expressions of spiritual need, therefore, may best be seen as giving patients an experience of God. By being present, by listening empathically, by responding in ways that foster increased self-awareness, HCPs are extending a sense of compassion, a taste of the sacred.

Guidelines

Several guidelines[5] for using helping skills are essential to observe:

1. *Be nondirective* (versus authoritarian) as a helper. Allow the solutions and answers to come from the patient. (An authoritarian helper gives lots of advice and interpretations, dominates the encounter, and allows little silence.)

2. *Keep the conversation ball in the patient's court* as much as possible. If a patient is talking productively, let him or her talk. When the patient stops (and silence won't be helpful) or begins talking aimlessly, then speak.

3. *Don't scratch where it doesn't itch.* That is, don't over-respond to distress by dramatizing it and don't introduce spiritual stressors that the patient has not yet introduced into conversation. For example, don't ask how someone answers the "why me?" question if he or she has not first implied that he or she has asked it.

4. *Focus on the core theme* when responding. While listening, ask yourself what is at the core of what the patient is saying. What is the main thought or feeling? What is key? What is it that the patient wants you to hear?

5. *Focus on the patient*, not on the pathology, the relatives, religious beliefs and practices, and so forth. Rather, focus on the patient's feelings about the pathology, the patient's perspective on the relatives, or the patient's religious experience.

6. *Focus on the present.* This includes how the past informs the present and how the present will affect the future.

7. *Use the patient's language style.* While it can be helpful to use the key words that he or she uses (especially labels for God, faith, and religious terms), try not to be a parrot who repeats phrases and sentences. This would show that you didn't try to understand what was said. For example:

RN: *How are you dealing with all this pain?*

PT: *My family helps, and my faith. [points upward]*

RN: *How does your faith help you? [a helpful response, in contrast with "How does Jesus help you?" when it is unknown if Jesus— or even God—is part of this patient's experience]*

8. *Vary the manner* with which you form your responses. For example, don't always begin with "You feel . . ." or "I hear you saying. . . ." Be human.

9. *Keep your responses short.* The micro-skills introduced in

this chapter usually require only a sentence of speech. Use words the patient will understand.

10. *Use the same sensory orientation of the patient.*[6] Although it is not essential, it may help you to connect better with the patient. Most people describe their experiences from a visual, auditory, or kinesthetic perspective. Try to use words that reflect that sensory orientation when responding. For example:

Visual

PT: *"It's hard for me to* see *how God could let this happen."*

MD: *"Tell me about how you* picture *God."*

Auditory

PT: *"I know this* sounds *bad, but can't God* hear *our cries for help?"*

HCP: *"It seems to you like God isn't* listening.*"*

Kinesthetic

PT: *"Why? I just wish I could* feel *God as a warm, loving* presence *right now."*

RN: *"It would be reassuring now if God would* touch *you in some loving way."*

11. *Talk heart to heart or head to head.* When do you use which micro-skill?

- If the patient is speaking from the "head" (e.g., telling a story, talking about ideas, facts), then give a head response (i.e., restatement, open question).

- If the patient is speaking from close to the "heart" (e.g., describing feelings deep within, soul searching), then respond to the heart with a reflection of feelings. Often, you will recognize speech from the heart because of the overt physical indicators that may accompany it, such as tears, a guttural voice, or a big sigh.

A patient who is talking from his head may be turned off by an HCP who responds with a reflection addressing the heart (feelings). Conversely, a patient who shares intimately from her heart about suffering will likely be disappointed and unaided by an HCP who asks her yet another question.

EXERCISE 5.2

Next to each HCP response, write down the numbers of the above guidelines that are *not* observed.

PT1: Why? Why did *I* get this disease? [strong emotion in voice, eyes tearing]

_____HCP1: Well, [deep breath] you're wondering what could explain getting this disease. We don't completely understand it yet. The research suggests . . .

PT2: You know, my dad used to say I was "human trash." Boy, he knew how to give a lickin' too! Yeah, it was tough growing up.

_____HCP2: So how did that used to make you feel? What else did he say to you?

PT3: I'm just praying that God will guide my surgeon's hands. I just can see his steady, caring hands there on Dr. Ahn's hands when I pray. It'll all turn out fine; there's no reason for me to be nervous. I'm just praying hard!

_____HCP3: Yes, and be sure you stay positive. I remember you telling me that it wasn't this way the last time you had surgery. I'm so glad you're sounding more optimistic this time. I'm sure Jesus will be with you and hear your prayers. Yes, Jesus has answered my prayers for health, too. Once I . . .

See "Answers for Exercises," page 132, for the best responses.

Micro-skill 1: Building rapport

The most important criteria patients have for a doctor or nurse who will discuss their spirituality is relationship.[7] More than their sharing similar spiritual beliefs, more than their having training in spiritual care, patients want HCPs to "just take a personal interest in me." Because HCPs typically do not have much time to develop relationships, it is fortunate that rapport can be built rapidly.

Tips for building rapport

Tips[8] for creating rapport rapidly include:

- Maintain comfortable eye contact that is at the same level as the patient (e.g., don't look down on the patient, don't prolong eye contact for those of cultures in which it is considered intrusive or disrespectful).

- Face the patient from a 90–180 degree angle, using body language that communicates openness (e.g., don't cross your arms) and cultural sensitivity.

- It is often helpful to match patients' body language, mood, and voice tone, speed, volume, and rhythm. This allows you to build a bridge to them so that you can understand them better.[9] Once you have matched a patient's emotional and physical posture, then you can gradually return him or her to a more comfortable state by modeling that state while you continue to interact with him or her.

- Comment on things that you appreciate about the patient or his or her belongings to offer an in-

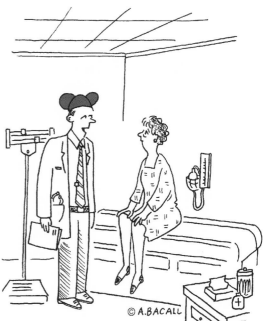

"I know the hat looks foolish but it shows that I'm all ears and interested in your concerns."

direct affirmation and show your personal interest. Experienced spiritual care clinician Wil Alexander takes this advice a step further and often opens a conversation with a new patient by asking, "For what are you famous?" These tips will help you to build rapport rapidly.

The stress of having a health challenge, however, also automatically increases a patient's sense of vulnerability and desire for your caring.

A story

Herta, a thirty-seven-year-old nurse from Germany, was studying in the United States when she was diagnosed with thyroid cancer. She tells this story of waiting for her thyroidectomy on a gurney in the operating room holding area:

I had said goodbye to my husband, and was wheeled into a huge waiting area. At that point, fear started to affect me. And my IV was really hurting. A nurse came, checked my name, birth date, and vitals, and then disappeared. Feeling chilly and alone, my level of anxiety rose. I silently prayed: "Lord, help me through this! This is the hour!" A few minutes later, another nurse approached my bed. He asked if I was comfortable or if I needed an additional warm blanket. I was grateful for the offer and told him that my IV was hurting. As he covered me with a warm blanket and changed something on my IV, he picked up on my German accent and started a very casual conversation with me about German football. In the midst of this conversation, I realized that my tension and fear had left. It was not a real deep conversation that did this, but how this nurse showed an interest in my immediate needs and chatted with me about the ordinary things of life. As short as the interaction was, it made such a difference! The first nurse never connected with me as a person, so I withdrew within myself. She just focused on the mechanics of her job, seemingly not seeing the person behind her work. The second nurse took an interest in who I was as a person. I must say,

if the first nurse had tried to pray with me or talk about spiritual-
ity, it would have seemed totally odd and displaced. With the sec-
ond nurse, however, this would have been an option! But even with-
out talking about spirituality or even praying, he touched my spirits
in a crucial moment and helped me cope—probably without being
aware of it!

EXERCISE 5.3

You enter the hospital room of a woman whom you've never
met before. You know she has just been diagnosed with a termi-
nal illness. You knock and hear her voice, muffled, a bit slow, and
sounding irritated. You find her curled up in a ball, eyes shut, cov-
ers pulled up to her ears. The lights are off and the shade is par-
tially drawn. How would you apply the above information about
establishing rapport?

_____

_____

_____

_____

See "Answers for Exercises," page 132, for one good response.

Micro-skill 2: Restatements

Restatements involve saying back a distilled version of what someone has said. A restatement is not only shorter, but also clearer
and more concrete than the original statement.[10] Restatements
are helpful when a patient is having difficulty focusing his or her
thoughts and needs help to hear what he or she is saying. The purpose of restatements is to clarify or focus a patient's thoughts (not
feelings). Restatements can summarize or paraphrase the present
or previous encounters.

Consider the following examples:

Mother whose eleven-year-old daughter has just been diagnosed with Type I diabetes mellitus: "My sweet Rosie! She was such a good girl. She has so much potential for the future, and now this! [crying] Why do bad things happen to innocent children?"

HCP: "Rosie's disease is bringing you to question why unfair and unjust things happen."

Patient with stage IV breast cancer: "I've prayed so hard to be healed. I've been sick for six years. I was diagnosed on my birthday, can you believe it? And prayed every day to God that He would take this sickness away. The Bible says he will heal all our diseases, you know. Maybe I'm praying in the wrong way."

HCP: "You've been fervently petitioning God to cure you, and now, perhaps, you're wondering if you're doing it in the right way."

An eighty-seven-year-old home care patient: "I've just had so many friends and family die in the last few months. I don't know how much I can stand. My brother-in-law, my sister, my hairdresser. And then my niece, that was especially hard to accept. I keep thinking maybe God is trying to teach me something, but I don't know what."

HCP: "It sounds as though while you grieve, you're pondering what God might be trying to teach you."

Tips for restating

How do you create a restatement? Here is advice:[11]

Assume you do not understand anything about the patient.
Your restatements are allowing you to learn what you can from the patient.

Pick the one most significant aspect of what the patient is saying to restate.

Cues that inform what is most significant include:

- noting nonverbal expressions (they are more honest than verbal ones);

- what topic the patient spends time and energy on;

- questions, conflicts, or unresolved issues the patient raises.

Keep the restatement short.

Even if it is a summary or a paraphrase, try to keep it to a sentence.

Use tentativeness.

Be careful so you don't offend the patient with certainty or inaccuracy. Tentative words, tone of voice, or facial expression allow a patient to feel comfortable correcting your observation if it is necessary. Phrases you can use include:

- "It sounds as though . . . "

- "I wonder if . . . "

- "Perhaps . . . "

If you really don't understand what the patient is trying to say, ask the patient to repeat the thought.

This is better than making a patient feel you didn't listen when you create a restatement that "misses the boat."

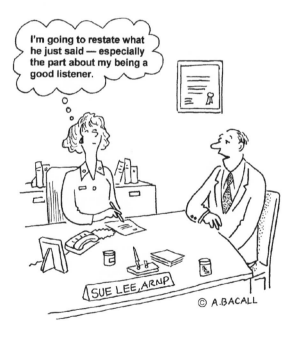

I'm going to restate what he just said — especially the part about my being a good listener.

SUE LEE, ARNP

© A. BACALL

Try your hand now at creating some restatements!

PT: "You know, I used to drink a lot. My wife would get mad at me. I'd just avoid her. Then I blew up like a volcano one night. I didn't mean to hurt her. I dunno. I just can't believe it all happened. It seems like a nightmare. It is a nightmare. I can't believe I did that—I just can't forgive myself."

YOU: _____

_____

_____

_____

_____

PT: "I was in the prime of life! Then the MS started to bother me. Why? Now I have to wear diapers. I can't make love. Nobody wants me."

YOU: _____

_____

_____

PT: "I hate not being able to take care of myself. My family says they don't mind. But that's the words. They act different-ly. I don't want to die. What is there for me to do now? Why should I live? I'm just a burden to others. Sometimes I'd just rather be dead."

YOU: _____

_____

_____

_____

_____

Check both the above general guidelines and the tips for making restatements. How do your restatements follow these recommendations? See also "Answers for Exercises," page 133.

Table 5.1 Indicators of the Effectiveness of a Restatement[12]

Ineffective restatements 1	Moderately ineffective or neutral restatements 2	Effective restatements 3
Patient stops exploring, gets frustrated, clams up.	Patient talks, but keeps repeating or "circling."	Patient elaborates further, introduces new aspects to topic, feels understood.

Table 5.1 summarizes indicators of effectiveness of a restatement. Imagine how a patient would respond to your restatements, and then rate them as a 1, 2, or 3.

Micro-skill 3: Open questions

Open questions are the opposite of closed questions, which allow only a "yes," "no," or short, factual answer. Open questions allow a patient to clarify and explore thoughts or feelings; they help a patient to consider "what's going on." Open questions are especially helpful when patients ask questions that are perplexing or intriguing. A helpful response could include: "Tell me more of your thoughts about this" or "What brought that question to mind [now]?"

Although open questions are extremely helpful tools, they are often overused. It is not unusual for HCPs to avoid emotional discomfort in a conversation by simply asking another question. Or, when HCPs don't know what to say next, they often use an open question as filler. Sometimes HCPs ask questions out of curiosity; these questions not only take up time, but steer the conversation away from the key concern. Bombarding a patient with questions can keep a conversation away from deeper feelings, allow the HCP to dominate the conversation, and put pressure on the patient to respond. Therefore, use open questions sparingly.

Consider these examples:

Mother whose eleven-year-old daughter has just been diagnosed with Type I diabetes mellitus: "My sweet Rosie! She was such a good girl. She has so much potential for the future, and now this! [crying] Why do bad things happen to innocent children?"

HCP: "You ask a deep question. What sorts of answers have you thought about?"

Patient with stage IV breast cancer: "I've prayed so hard to be healed. I've been sick for six years. I was diagnosed on my birthday, can you believe it? And prayed every day to God that he would take this sickness away. The Bible says he will heal all our diseases, you know. Maybe I'm praying in the wrong way."

HCP: "Tell me about what praying the right way might be like?"

An eighty-seven-year-old home care patient: "I've just had so many friends and family die in the last few months. I don't know how much I can stand. My brother-in-law, my sister, my hairdresser. And then my niece, that was especially hard to accept. I keep thinking maybe God is trying to teach me something, but I don't know what."

HCP: "How do you think God is thinking right now?"

Tips for asking open questions

The following tips[13] can assist you to effectively use open questions in response to patients' expressions of spiritual distress:

Before asking, consider: "Will the question I want to ask be helpful to the patient?" Ask no more than two open questions in a row.

Asking too many open questions may be an indicator of your discomfort or need to control the conversation. An alternative to asking a question is to rephrase your question into a restatement or reflection. For example, rather than ask, "Are you worried about being a burden to your family?" you can state, "I sense you are worried about being a burden to your family."

Often a restatement or reflection is uncomfortable to offer, so the professional adds a questioning inflection at the end of the statement. You can avoid this tendency simply by becoming aware of the habit. For example, instead of "You're feeling _____?" just say "It seems like you're feeling _____."

Ask about "hows" and "whats."

Avoid asking "why" questions, as they are threatening.

Vary the way you ask questions.

For example, don't always start with "So what do you think/feel about . . . ?" and don't always follow-up with "What do you mean?" Other good ways to begin an open question include: "Tell me more about . . . ," "Give me an example of . . . ," or "Explain . . ."

Ask one question at a time.

Refrain from questions where the answer is implied.

It is condescending. For example, "You don't really believe that, do you?" Not only is this a yes/no question, it suggests the answer.

Avoid sounding interrogative or judgmental.

Instead, use a tone of voice that conveys sincere compassion. (And remember, you really can't fake compassion!) You can also avoid quizzing by asking a question indirectly. For example, ask "I wonder how it feels to . . . ?" instead of "How does it feel . . . ?"

Don't implore or coerce a patient to answer a question.

Refusal to answer or a shallow answer is also information. The patient may not want to talk about the topic or may not want to talk about it with you. You may respond with a restatement about what you are observing and offer a way you can care, if it is appropriate. For example, "I'm sensing that you don't feel like talking right now. Know that I care" [pause, and move on]. Or, "Perhaps this topic is very tiring. If you'd like to talk to me or a spiritual care expert later, let me or one of the other team members know so we can arrange it."

EXERCISE 5.5

Try your hand now at creating some open questions!

PT: "You know, I used to drink a lot. My wife would get mad at me. I'd just avoid her. Then I blew up like a volcano one night. I didn't mean to hurt her. I dunno. I just can't believe it all happened. It seems like a nightmare. It is a nightmare. I can't believe I did that—I just can't forgive myself."

YOU: _____

_____

PT: "I was in the prime of life! Then the MS started to bother me. Why? Now I have to wear diapers. I can't make love. Nobody wants me."

YOU: _____

_____

PT: "I hate not being able to take care of myself. My family says they don't mind. But that's the words. They act differently. I don't want to die. What is there for me to do now? Why should I live? I'm just a burden to others. Sometimes I'd just rather be dead."

YOU: _____

_____

Check both the above general guidelines and the tips for asking open question. How do your open questions follow these recommendations? See also "Answers for Exercises," page 133.

Table 5.2 Indicators of the Effectiveness of an Open Question[14]

Ineffective open questions 1	Moderately effective open questions 2	Effective open questions 3
Patient gives minimal response to question; may show annoyance, anger.	Patient continues to talk, but repeating or "circling." says the same things over again, indicating no new clarity or understanding.	Patient delves deeper into issue, may reveal more information about thoughts, feelings related to issue.

Table 5.2 summarizes indicators of effectiveness of an open question. Imagine how a patient would respond to your questions, and then rate them as a 1, 2, or 3.

Micro-skill 4: Reflecting feelings and advanced empathy

"Emotions belong at the center of spirituality, not at its edges. . . . [F]eelings often provide a powerful window to the Holy."[15] Feelings inform us; they are an approach to knowing. Helping patients to recognize their feelings, therefore, is another way HCPs can support spiritual healing.

Reflecting feelings involves restating what feelings a patient has expressed verbally or nonverbally. While it typically takes several words or phrases to describe a thought, it usually takes only one word to describe a feeling.[16] Reflecting feelings allows you to show empathy and understanding. Being able to name overt and, especially, covert, deep feelings is the fundamental component of an empathic response.[17]

Psychologists Hill and O'Brien explain why reflecting feelings is an essential micro-skill for helpers:

Often we ignore, deny, distort, or repress our feelings because we have been told that they are unacceptable. Hence, we grow apart from our inner experiencing and cannot accept ourselves. We need to return to our emotions and allow ourselves to feel them because only then can we decide what we want to do about them.[18]

A healing response for patients is one that gives compassion. You will give compassion by understanding their feelings and offering them an opportunity to recognize these feelings.

Consider these examples:

Mother whose eleven-year-old daughter has just been diagnosed with Type I diabetes mellitus): "My sweet Rosie! She was such a good girl. She has so much potential for the future, and now this! [crying] Why do bad things happen to innocent children?"

HCP: "It seems that you're angry because a future is shattered."

Patient with stage IV breast cancer: "I've prayed so hard to be healed. I've been sick for six years. I was diagnosed on my birthday, can you believe it? And prayed every day to God that he would take this sickness away. The Bible says he will heal all our diseases, you know. Maybe I'm praying in the wrong way."

HCP: "You're frustrated, maybe, about how to relate to God."

An eighty-seven–year-old home care patient: "I've just had so many friends and family die in the last few months. I don't know how much I can stand. My brother-in-law, my sister, my hairdresser. And then my niece, that was especially hard to accept. I keep thinking maybe God is trying to teach me something, but I don't know what."

HCP: "I'm guessing you're feeling bewildered."

Tips for reflecting feelings

The following tips[19] can assist you to use feeling reflections effectively in response to patients' expressions of spiritual distress:

Ask, "How would I feel given this situation if I were from this culture, social class, and family?"

Although you do not want to project or impose your feelings onto patients, you can begin to recognize their feelings by noticing their feeling words and nonverbal indicators of feeling.

When forming a response, try to match both feeling type and intensity.

There are two aspects to naming a feeling: 1) what type of feeling (e.g., sad, glad, mad, bad); and 2) intensity of the feeling.

- For patients who are likely defensive about their feelings (and most of us are—especially with negative feelings!), err on underrating intensity. For example, anger can range from mild irritation or frustration to intense fury. A patient who may have difficulty admitting anger may be approached best with a reflection such as, "Perhaps you're frustrated because . . ."

- When you are proficient at making feeling reflections, you may describe the intensity of the patient's feelings with near accuracy, even though the patient is unready to recognize this intensity. You will be leading him or her towards naming the feeling he or she is just becoming aware of.

- *At first, use the beginner's recipe for reflecting feelings: "You feel _____ because (or when) _____."* This can be abbreviated by saying: "You feel _____." This recipe, however, can make responses sound unnatural. As you become more proficient, drop the recipe and express your empathy in your own unique way while naming the feeling (see Table 5.3).

Table 5.3 Four Ways of Stating a Reflection of Feelings[20]

Type of feeling reflection	Description	Examples
Single word	Feeling is described by one word.	"I can tell you're really relieved." "You're disappointed." "It seems you're feeling tense."
Phrase	A phrase or metaphor that describes the feeling.	"You're feeling like a helpless baby." "You have 'cabin fever.'" "You feel like a sailboat without a sail."
Experiential statement	A statement that implies the feeling. It uses the part of the beginner's recipe that comes after the "because."	"You feel part of you has died" [implies feeling of grief]; "You feel like nobody cares" [implies feeling of abandonment].
Behavioral statement	Feeling is implied by stating what action the patient feels like taking.	"You feel like throwing in the towel" [implied feeling of futility or despair]; "You feel like never letting go of your kids" [implied feeling of fear].

Recognize that reflecting feelings, or helping the patient to become more aware of inner feelings, is a process.

The process involves making tentative reflections, allowing the patient to circle around the targeted feeling, correcting and fine-tuning the feeling. For example:

HCP: "I'm wondering if you're feeling a little blue because you got some bad news today."

PT: "Actually, the news makes me really depressed!"

HCP: "Oh, I'm guessing you feel really depressed because the news makes you angry about how your body is going to change."

PT: "Well, more because I'm just so sad. I'm not going to be able to do all those things that make my life seem worth living."

HCP: [after thoughtful pause to let ideas sink in, speaks tentatively] "You're sad because what brought you pleasure and purpose is being taken from you."

PT: "Now that you put it that way, yeah, and it also [expletive deleted] me off. Hell, I am angry, too!"

Be tentative and cautious as you introduce a reflection of feelings.

There is great potential for hurting patients by imposing an observation about their feelings. After all, you do not know exactly what the patient is feeling. Use a gentle tone of voice. Use words that indicate your reflection is a hunch and that you still have some doubt about the accuracy of your reflection (e.g., I gather . . . , If I'm hearing you correctly . . . , I'm wondering if you are feeling . . . ," or "I'm not sure, maybe you're feeling . . . ," or "I'd venture that you're feeling . . .").

Do not use feeling reflections if the patient is not ready to listen.

Although reflection of feelings is a very powerful tool, do not use feeling reflections when the patient is having a severe emotional crisis (or has a history of dealing poorly with emotional crises) or when he or she shows strong resistance to talking about feelings.

Accept tears as a sign of healing.

Feelings and matters of the heart are often buried deep within. When you uncover them, they may be accompanied by tears (perhaps nature's washing out the dust or cobwebs). What is often most helpful during times of fresh tears is silent presence.

When you miss the mark and fail to name the feeling the patient is experiencing, do not apologize.

Rather, try again to hone in on the feeling. You can say something such as, "I didn't understand you very well; can you tell me more about what you are feeling?"

When a patient agrees with your reflection but fails to explore the feeling further, pause to allow time for the observation to sink in.

If necessary, you can follow up with a statement such as, "Perhaps you're unsure of what to do with this inner experience/feeling."

Try your hand now at creating some reflections for feelings!

PT: "You know, I used to drink a lot. My wife would get mad at me. I'd just avoid her. Then I blew up like a volcano one night. I didn't mean to hurt her. I dunno. I just can't believe it all happened. It seems like a nightmare. It is a nightmare. I can't believe I did that—I just can't forgive myself."

YOU: _____

_____

_____

_____

PT: "I was in the prime of life! Then the MS started to bother me. Why? Now I have to wear diapers. I can't make love. Nobody wants me. Why? I don't know what I'm going to do. Why is this happening to me?"

YOU: _____

_____

_____

_____

PT: "I hate not being able to take care of myself. My family says they don't mind. But that's the words. They act differently. I don't want to die. What is there for me to do now? Why should I live? I'm just a burden to others. Sometimes I just rather be dead."

YOU: _____

_____

_____

_____

Table 5.4 Indicators of the Effectiveness of Feeling Reflections[21]

Ineffective reflection 1	Moderately effective reflection 2	Effective reflection 3
Patient responses to inaccurate and ill-timed reflections include: disagreeing, changing or ignoring the subject, disengaging from clinician, becoming angry or defensive, giving a superficial response. Ultimately, if there is no exploration of feelings, the reflection was ineffective.	Patient may agree with reflection, but does not explore further; may talk more, but not about feelings. May show a release of some emotion.	Patient may verbally or non-verbally agree; explores self and world deeply, gaining new insight; releases emotion (e.g., sighs, cries).

Check both the above general guidelines and the tips for reflecting feelings. How do your open questions follow these recommendations? For example, do your reflections:

□ *Focus on the patient and the present?*

□ *Focus on the core theme or issue, the spiritual need?*

□ *Approximately match the patient's feeling, including the intensity of that feeling?*

Table 5.4 summarizes indicators of effectiveness of feeling reflections. Imagine how a patient would respond to your questions and rate them as 1, 2, or 3.

EXERCISE 5.7

Consider this scenario and write four feeling reflections, one for each type described in Table 5.3.

A father of a twenty-five-year-old son who has just been given two weeks to live: "'My God, my God, why have you forsaken me?' That's what Jesus said on the cross and that's what I'm saying every moment. My heart is breaking. I'd rather it be me dying. A son isn't supposed to die before his father! [tears]"

Single word: _____

Phrase: _____

Experiential statement: _____

_____

Behavioral statement: _____

_____

See "Answers for Exercises," page 133.

Advanced empathy

You have now learned the basics of how to reflect feelings. What is most healing, however, is not only identifying the key feeling, but naming the deeper, often hidden feeling. When this is done, the patient is encouraged to:

- See the bigger picture (e.g., "Maybe you're mad not just at people at your temple, but also at God").

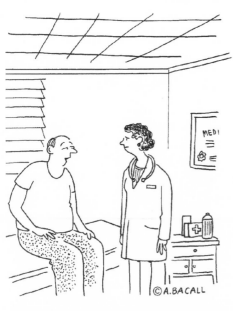

"You're a very good listener. You hear my feelings."

- Hear what he or she is implying or hinting about (e.g., "I'm wondering if what I hear in your 'why?' is also a question about if God exists").

- Draw a logical conclusion from what he or she is saying (e.g., "From our conversation, it seems that maybe you're exhausted by this disease and ready to pass on").

- Identify what the patient may be avoiding or overlooking (e.g., death, anger, religious doubt).

- Recognize a theme in what they are saying (e.g., "You've mentioned several times now, if I remember right, that you're afraid of sinning and going to hell").

- Own their partly verbalized experiences, behaviors, and feelings (e.g., "You've mentioned being frustrated by how your stoma is going to affect you. I'm wondering if there isn't some pretty strong anger deep inside about it").[22]

To unearth the deeper feelings of a patient, therefore, an HCP must privately ask:

What is the patient only half saying?
At what is the patient hinting?
What is the patient saying in a confused way?
What feelings do the postural and non-verbal messages convey?[23]

Carkhuff[24] described clinicians' empathic responses by levels or degrees of effectiveness (see Table 5.5). Whereas levels 1 and 2 responses are not effective, levels 3-5 responses are healing. Although level 5 responses are extremely effective, they are overwhelming when used frequently. Hammond and colleagues[25] recommend that helpers mostly use level 3 responses, and occasionally interject level 4 or 5 empathic responses. Level 4 or 5 reflections can even be un-

Table 5.5 Carkhuff's Levels of Empathic Response[26]

Carkhuff level of empathic response	Description
Level 1 [unhelpful]	Helper is not listening, shows no awareness of patient's feelings.
Level 2 [unhelpful]	Helper has awareness of the most superficial feelings expressed by the patient; responses fail to recognize these feelings, however. Responses often avoid or minimize the patient's painful feelings.
Level 3	Helper's responses match the surface feelings expressed by the patient.
Levels 4 and 5	Helper's responses recognize the deeper feeling and its meaning, integrate feeling and thinking. Because the helper is fully tuned in to the patient's feelings, the patient is helped to explore the depth of his feelings—feelings of which he or she is minimally aware—more than before.

helpful unless the following are in place: a trusting patient-clinician relationship, patient is indicating positive feelings toward the HCP, the patient is taking initiative to explore self and become more self-aware, and level 3 responses have been effective just prior to this deeper reflection.

EXERCISE 5.8

Using Carkhuff's levels of empathy, match the level of empathy with illustrative response to the following scenario:

An eight-month-old with "shaken baby syndrome" caused by the mother's boyfriend is on a ventilator in a pediatric intensive care unit. The mother is visiting and caressing the baby. She turns to you, sobbing, and says, "I am not a bad mom. I never thought this would happen. I shouldn't have left her. I shouldn't have trusted him. If only I hadn't moved in with him . . ."

Level of empathic response	Illustrative response to mother
Level 1: _____	a. "It makes you really mad. You wish you could replay the past."
Level 2: _____	b. "OK, let's check and see how her lungs sound now."
Level 3: _____	c. "You never know who you can trust these days. At least he didn't kill her."
Level 4/5: _____	d. "Sounds like you're not only mad at your boyfriend, but maybe also at yourself for leaving your baby with him."

See "Answers to Exercises," page 134.

EXERCISE 5.9

After the following scenarios, write reflections that illustrate both basic and advanced empathy.

Case 1

A retired physician with end-stage renal disease is dying. He has been active in his church since childhood. After his minister and leaders of his church conduct an anointing ritual intended to petition God for healing, this physician (PT) confides to you (HCP):

PT: I don't think it will do any good.

HCP: Tell me what you mean.

PT: Well, you know, I am definitely dying. There's no changing that. God doesn't violate his own laws of nature. I need to just accept the fact that I'm dying. [pause] But I sure wish God would heal me. I got to admit, the fact that he doesn't sure stretches my faith to the breaking point.

HCP: [What would you say?]

Basic empathic response (What feeling most requires attention? What is the intensity of this feeling?):

_____

_____

_____

_____

Advanced empathic response (What is below the surface here? What is being avoided and hinted?):

_____

_____

_____

Case 2

The wife of a ventilated patient with a grim prognosis says:

WIFE: He's going to get well. The doctor says so!

HCP: I sense your desperation about wanting your husband to get well.

WIFE: [begins to tear] Oh, I just can't imagine life without him. What would I do? He can't die! What am I going to do if he dies?

HCP: [What would you say?]

Basic empathic response:

_____

_____

Advanced empathic response:

_____

_____

See "Answers for Exercises," page 134.

Micro-skill 5: Self-disclosure

"Nurse, do you believe in prayer?" "Doc, what happens after we die?" "What do you believe?" HCPs get such questions from patients. Answering such questions for a patient requires self-disclosure, or talking about yourself. You are, after all, a fellow traveler along the road of life. You likely not only share with the patient spiritual questions and doubts, but also satisfying spiritual perspectives and ways of finding comfort. You can model spiritual sensitivity and awareness. Principles about how to use self-disclosure for therapeutic purposes should guide HCPs' responses to such queries.

Tips for using self-disclosure

When self-disclosing personal spiritual perspectives, the HCP can maintain a therapeutic relationship with the patient by remembering the following:[27]

Do not disclose to gratify your needs.

Ask yourself, "Whose needs are being met when I share my beliefs?" If you are disclosing your beliefs because you think they will benefit the patient, yet the patient has no desire to know your beliefs, then you are meeting your needs. Asking a patient if you can share your beliefs may be inappropriate, given that patients often perceive they are "at your mercy" and may feel uncomfortable declining your offer.

When patients ask you about your spirituality, you may find it helpful to first assess why they are asking.

For example, "Your question about _____ is a tough one. What brings you to ask it now?" Or, "I love talking about my beliefs, but what in particular is it that you'd like to know?" Or, "Before I answer, could we explore what this means to you?" The *why* behind the question should guide your response. While many patients are looking for explanations or beliefs that will satisfy their questions, others may simply be curious or wanting to equalize their relationship with you by reciprocating an interest in your personal life. They may also want to check to see if you share similar beliefs, a prerequisite for some who want to discuss their spirituality. More covert meanings behind such inquiries can include: Will you judge me? Are you safe?

Any time you disclose your personal beliefs, follow up the self-disclosure with an open question or reflection of feelings.

Always return the ball to the patient's court. For example, "As you can see, I'm not sure of this myself, but can you tell me what would be comforting to you?" Or, "I wonder what is going on inside you now?" You may also preface your self-disclosure with a statement such as, "I want to answer, but then I'd like to hear what you feel about what I have to say."

Use self-disclosure infrequently and keep the disclosures short.

A request about what you believe is not a request for a lesson from your sacred scripture or your complete spiritual history.

Keep your answer honest, authentic.

Sometimes this means simply saying, "I don't know."

If you are asked a question you are uncomfortable with or are unable to answer, you can still use the moment for healing purposes.

Healing can still occur when you use the micro-skills introduced above to increase self-awareness. For example, "You know, I have to admit, I'm uncomfortable with your question. I may be uncomfortable with it because I don't like the answers I've heard others give for it. Perhaps asking the question makes you feel uncomfortable, too." [pause for response] Or, "I've been wondering that myself for a long time. Sometimes I wonder if it is . . . , but I don't know. What ideas have you considered?" With the patient's permission, make a referral to a trained chaplain or the patient's clergy.

EXERCISE 5.10

Create helpful self-disclosing responses for the following:

Patient receiving dialysis for end-stage renal disease asks: "Do you think there is a life after death?"

YOU: _____

_____

_____

_____

Mother of a twenty-six-year-old man with depression who committed suicide: "My church teaches that suicide is a sin. But my son was suffering so much. How could God hold this against my son? Tell me, I really want an answer!"

YOU: _____

_____

_____

_____

Terminally ill patient with unmanageable pain: "What good could possibly come from this experience? What could God be thinking, anyway? Yes, I do want to know what you think."

YOU: _____

_____

_____

_____

Check both the above general guidelines and the tips for self-disclosure. Do your self-disclosures follow these recommendations?

□ *Is your response trying to meet the patient's need or yours?*

□ *Is your response short?*

□ *Is your response honest?*

□ *Does your response place the ball in the patient's court?*

Table 5.6 summarizes indicators of effectiveness of a self-disclosure. Imagine how a patient would respond to your self-disclosures and rate them as a 1, 2, or 3.

Table 5.6 Indicators of the Effectiveness of Self-Disclosure[28]

Ineffective self-disclosure 1	Moderately effective self-disclosure 2	Effective self-disclosure 3
Patient responds by trying to end conversation, shows anger for having been "preached" to, or fails to further explore beliefs or feelings. Therapeutic relationship is breached.	Patient does not explore further; may talk more, but not about feelings or deeper significance of personal questions, doubts. Relationship is not stressed.	Patient may quietly reflect further, or explore beliefs and feeling more deeply, gaining new insight. Relationship may become more intimate, yet remains professional.

EXERCISE 5.11

Return to Exercise 1.1 (at the end of chapter one). Now formulate two possible responses for the scenario, including a reflection of the deeper feeling present.

1._____

_____

2._____

_____

Review the pertinent tips to see if you followed directions. How well did you do? If you had been this patient, how would you react to these responses? Would there be greater insight? A sigh of relief?

6 Verbal Responses to Spiritual Pain

Macro-skills

Now that you have learned to use the micro-skills of chapter five, you can blend and build on those skills while you apply the "macro-skills" presented in this chapter. These approaches are more complex and require more perspective on a patient's spirituality. These macro-skills, or spiritual care therapeutics, include story listening, body listening, promoting resilience and reframing, and supporting helpful religious practices.

Although this book is focused on patients with spiritual needs and pain, it is important to remember that patients concurrently have spiritual strengths. All of the approaches presented in this chapter allow patients to become more aware of their ever-present spiritual assets.

Macro-skill 1: Story listening

Patients tell stories. These stories come in diverse forms, such as those that begin: "Once when I was young," "You know what just happened," or "A favorite book of mine tells the story of." Whether the stories are literal or figurative (and literal stories can be metaphorical), storytelling and reminiscence can promote spiritual healing.[1]

Why? Telling their stories helps patients transmit their legacies and values to others (providing a sense of purpose); helps them discover and better understand who they are (allowing them to weave together the disparate pieces of their lives to give it meaning); helps them build a warm connection to the listener; and helps them value the lives they have lived.[2]

For some patients, stories are the only way that they can express their feelings. Some patients may not have language for describing how they feel; they may be thinkers, not feelers. To allow such patients to access and express their inner experience the HCP must encourage and respond to their stories.

Tips for story listening

"In the telling of their stories, strangers befriend not only their host but also their own past."[3] The following tips will help you to be a gracious host(ess) that helps patients' to find meaning in their stories:[4]

Appreciate that every storyteller needs a listener.
Storytelling cannot serve its function unless someone listens carefully.

Remember the adage, "Chief complaint: No one will listen to my story."
It also explains why some patients repeat their stories, or pieces of their life story. The exasperation you may experience from listening to a story over and over can be lessened by remembering that it may be due to the patient not feeling heard. Indeed, stories get repeated when patients have not yet heard themselves speaking enough to make sense of their story.

Let patients tell their story in whatever way they choose.

Indeed, how they choose to tell their story is extremely informative. Avoid interrupting and forcing a story into a formula. You may observe, as did Kane,[5] that illness stories typically follow a pattern of devastation, reflection, and response.

Help patients connect their story to the present if they are unable.

For example, "I think I can see now why you told me that story; is what happened to you then like what's happening now?"

Assist patients to gain further self-understanding from their story by doing a "story check."

For example: "Your telling me the legend of Prometheus makes me wonder how you see yourself being like him." "How is the story you've just told me a lesson for your life?" "The stories you've been telling me about your life seem to have a theme about . . . Can you tell me more about that?" "I've learned from your story that you value . . . How does that help you now?" Ultimately, however, only the patient can interpret the story.

To gain perspective, privately consider questions that will help you to analyze the story.

For example:

- What is the storyteller choosing to remember, to forget? How self-deceptive or self-accepting is the teller?

- What values and beliefs are revealed in this story?

- What life themes emerge?

- How does the past influence the present?

- What unresolved conflicts surface?

- Is the story of illness chaotic or coherent? Is the patient able to ascribe meaning, connectedness with others, and hope to the personal suffering told in the story?

- For what might the story be a metaphor?
- Why was the story told now?
- How does the patient portray him- or herself (as a martyr, warrior, victim, or hero)?

As needed, help patients to place their stories within a redeeming or meaningful context.

For example, ask: "This is your life so far. How would you like the story to end?" (And, "What will it take for you to achieve that 'happily ever after' ending?") "Although you've had a lot of rough times in your life, what are the good things that have come from them?" "I heard you say that the bad things happened in your story because of . . . , but what other reasons might there be?" "How have all these _____ (e.g., losses) in your life helped to make you who you are—or how can you use them to make you the _____ (e.g., joyful) person you want to be?"

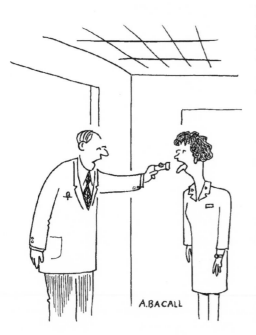

"It's nothing to worry about nurse. It's only teeth bites on your tongue. Lots of good listeners have them."

Recognize that you will have a counter-story.

Hearing another's story will undoubtedly evoke memories of your experience. Keep your story to yourself, or tell it to your friends, family, or therapist. While your story is essential to express, it usually is inappropriate to do so in response to a patient's storytelling (see chapter five, Self-disclosure).

Create healing responses to the following scenarios. Don't forget to use your micro-skills!

Case 1

Alice, a lucid, minimally demented ninety-three-year-old SNF resident, is telling you the following story, which you have heard several times before. She has received a thorough medical evaluation, which determined that there was no physical evidence of trauma from a fall that occurred two months prior.

My head hurts! [offered analgesic] No, I don't want medicine. I just wish they hadn't let me fall. I fell over here while I was coming from the bathroom in the middle of the night and I fell here and hit my head on the corner of my bed. Ow! It's like they don't care around here. I wish someone would do something. I need help. Help! Help! Yeah, I just fell down here and hit my head on the corner of the bed here. My head hurts. Can't someone do something?

Your response:_____
_____
_____
_____

Case 2

Ken is a thirty-five-year-old rehabilitation patient who is a war veteran:

[Expletive] this amputation sucks. If I hadn't been at that intersection at that exact moment, it wouldn't have been me. It wouldn't have been my leg. Reminds me of when I was in Iraq and my best buddy got killed in "friendly fire." You know, it's just not fair. We were patrolling in this desert region near the border. We were being really careful, watching for mines and stuff. The locals didn't seem too dangerous, we weren't that worried about them. And we were

both about to return home, in twenty-nine days for Tom, thirty-four for me. It's a clear, warm day, pretty nice. It's like it was yesterday. Then out of nowhere one of our F-14s comes over us, and [expletive] breaks loose! We both go down, but only Tom gets killed, instantly. It could have just as easily been me. [Expletive].

Your response: _____

_____

_____

_____

See "Answers for Exercises," page 134.

Macro-skill 2: Body listening

Although religious traditions have taught for centuries that the physical body houses the spirit, little attention is paid to how spiritual awareness can increase by listening to the body. Decades ago, Gendlin observed that successful psychotherapy patients had a special awareness of their internal body, whereas unsuccessful patients did not.[6] As a result of this research, the experiential focusing method was developed. It is used today to facilitate psychospiritual growth.

Tips for helping patients with body listening

The six steps of the focusing method that allow a patient to listen to the body's messages are presented in Table 6.1.[7] These six steps, however, take time and are cumbersome for the harried health care professional (HCP) and the distracted patient. Principles of focusing, however, can often be implemented. When a patient describes a spiritual concern, he or she can be encouraged to find a "handle," to name how this concern feels in his or her body. The patient can then be prompted with open questions so that he or she can explore the message of this bodily sensation. A patient can privately reflect on such questions long after the HCP has left.

Table 6.1 Steps for Body Listening[8]

Steps	Description	Questions to ask (examples)
1. Clear space.	Encourage the patient to consider what is on his or her list of concerns, and put all but one of these concerns aside.	"What's between you and feeling fine?"
2. Get a "felt sense."	Explore how this concern feels in the body.	"What do you sense in your body when you think about this concern?"
	Explore the qualities and location of this felt sense. Explore this sense as completely as possible, even the vagueness and unclear sense of it.	"What color, shape, or weight is it? Where is it centered?"
3. Get a "handle."	A handle is an image, word, or phrase to label and describe this sense. For example, a felt sense could be described as a "brown, heavy pressure on the chest," or "hollowness," or "jumping up and down."	"What word or picture would best capture or describe this sense in your body?"
4. Resonate.	Move between the handle and the felt sense to verify that they match. If they match, one is to focus on the experience of this matching several times. If the felt sense changes, one is to remain attentive to it.	"Tune in to that way your body feels about [name the concern]. Then, think about your handle. Go back and forth between these. How well do they seem to match up?"
5. Ask the felt sense an open question.	This allows understanding of its meaning. When insight occurs, a "felt shift" occurs (like when you finally remember where you put your keys). This "aha" moment brings relief, release, psycho-spiritual growth, renewed energy—healing. The felt shift is a grace; it cannot be forced. Through-out this process of asking, the patient must be reminded to "let the body answer." Allowing silence for inner awareness to occur is vital. The patient will need to look away or close his or her eyes to focus.	Three types of questions that explore the felt sense are: 1. General questions that ask about the felt sense (e.g., "What is that whole feeling about?" "What is it about this concern that feels ____?" "If this whole feeling could talk, what would it say?"). 2. Crux questions that focus on the heart of the concern, that dig deeper (e.g., "What is [the handle]-est about this whole concern?" "What's the crux of this whole thing for you?"). 3. "Felt shift" questions are asked to encourage the felt sense to shift, to encourage the psycho-spiritual awareness that comes from increased awareness of the body's feelings (e.g., "What does it need?" "How would it feel if it were all okay?").
6. Receive the felt shift.	Welcoming the insight from the bodily feeling is important, as it needs to be valued and integrated.	"How would you like to welcome this gift from your body?"

Suggest a response that will help this family caregiver (FCG) experience a "felt shift" (or that "aha" from finding meaning from a physical sensation).

FCG: I'm just so worried about him. He doesn't eat. He doesn't want to get out of bed. He just doesn't really seem to want to live. It makes me mad! Hey, why doesn't he want to make the most of what he's got? I just don't understand him.

YOU: You're pretty disappointed about his attitude toward living, it seems.

FCG: Exactly. And exasperated!

YOU: Yes, and at your wit's end about what to do. Maybe angry.

FCG: Yeah. I guess I should stop trying to want him to be somebody he's not. It's just leaving me angry.

YOU: Sounds like you're ready to see this as your issue, not his. [pause] Marie, how does this anger feel in your body?

FCG: Oh, it's just like there's this big lumpy, heavy ball in the pit of my stomach.

YOU: As you think about your anger, you get a feeling of a heavy ball in your stomach.

What would you ask next?

_____

_____

See "Answers for Exercises," page 135.

Macro-skill 3: Nurturing resilience and reframing

Resilience

Nurturing resilience involves transformation, a transforming of despair to hope, helplessness to empowerment, meaninglessness to meaningfulness, isolation to communion, resentment to grati-

tude, and sorrow to joy.[9] Numerous studies of seriously ill or traumatized persons directly link finding benefits from the illness with
psychological adaptation and spiritual growth,[10] and even physio-
logic adaptation.[11] Assisting patients to find the good in something
bad, therefore, is an appropriate goal for HCPs. To find the good
means one is resilient and able to mentally reframe the bad so that
it is also perceived as good. Not only does this process often tap
spiritual beliefs, it is spiritually healing.

Tips for nurturing resilience

Although HCPs cannot wave a magic wand to bring about such
transformation, they can ask open questions that encourage reflection and the transformation process. Types of questions that
nurture resilience include those about:

- Previous positive coping resources (e.g., "Have you ever
  had a tragedy in your life before this?" "What helped you
  through it?" "How could you use those strategies now?")

- Models to emulate (e.g., "What story about a hero facing the
  odds is your favorite?" "Who do you wish to be like most?"
  "How do you think he or she would face your challenge?"
  "How do you think you could be true to who you are and
  still be like this hero?")

- The specific state of vulnerability to counter, such as:

  Isolation (e.g., "Who suffers with you?" "Who do you feel saf-
  est talking to?" "How does God keep you company?")

  Despair (e.g., "Where do you find hope?" "When the going
  gets tough, what keeps you going?" "Who would expect you to
  be hopeful now?" "What do they know about you that others
  don't?")

  Helplessness (e.g., "Where do you get strength?" "What helps
  you the most now?" "How have you kept this illness from over-
  powering you?")

Meaninglessness (e.g., "For whom, or for what, do you still live?" "What do you want to accomplish with the life you still have?")

Sorrow, loss (e.g., "What helps you to still find joy amidst the sadness?" "What phoenixes have arisen from this loss?")

Resentment (e.g., "For what are you most thankful?")[12]

- Potential meaningful outcomes,[13] including perceived changes in

Self (e.g., "What has this illness taught you about yourself?")

Relationships with others (e.g., "How has your tragedy affected the way you relate to others now?")

Spirituality or philosophy of life (e.g., "How has this experience made you more in tune spiritually?" "How has it affected your sense of God?" "How has this experience clarified your beliefs?")

- Limit metaphors that are unhelpful or discomforting.[14] For example, "You mentioned that pain was something to 'just grin and bear' [or 'an enemy to fight' or 'a punishment']; can you think of other ways to relate to your pain?" Or, for a patient with a narrow view of God, "When you feel happy, what does your picture of God look like? And how does that compare with the picture you have now?"

Reframing

A quick way to form an attitude of gratitude is to choose a positive frame for a problem. The classic illustration of positive reframing is when a person thinks of a glass half full instead of half empty. Or, consider the Afghan metaphor of asking a candle, "Why do you burn?" The answer is, "I burn [cry, suffer] to give off my light."[15] Patients who are able to meaningfully reframe their suffering have more positive health outcomes.[16] For example, people with cancer who choose to view their pain as a challenge rather than an enemy, punishment, or other negative frame have less depression and pain.[17]

Tips for helping patients reframe

For an HCP to impose positivity on a patient's suffering is unhelpful, even destructive to a therapeutic relationship (see chapter two). It often is a way of avoiding a patient's suffering. Suggest positive frames for patients only when you know they will agree with them, or when you offer them tentatively in a question. The following tips on how to create positive frames for patients' "problems" heed this caution.[18]

Use downward comparison to compare with worse scenarios.

For example, "What I think I hear you saying is that you're glad you are not as sick as . . ." or "I'm imagining that you're thankful this happened now instead of earlier when . . . [e.g., your kids were young; when doctors couldn't treat this disease]." Or, in reverse, (if congruent with beliefs), "This life of living with rheumatoid arthritis is so short compared to the pain-free eternal life that is to come."

Consider how the "problem" is a good thing in another context.

Give the problem a new interpretation or spin. For example, "Perhaps this forced bed rest is an opportunity to get in touch with your creativity more?" Or, "It seems that this isolation has been good in that you've been forced to do some soul searching." Or, "Just think, you might not have been so honest with God ("angry") if you hadn't had this 'wake-up call' (pain) from your body." Thus, doubt can be a tool for exploring faith, rejecting one's religious past can be a statement about becoming spiritually congruent, feeling inwardly restless or lonely can be a homing instinct or yearning for God, and so forth. Fears can help us by informing us of danger. Grief reminds us of attachments for which we're grateful. Anger is a source of energy.

Notice and compliment the patient's strengths.

For example, "I am so impressed with your perseverance. You could have chosen a lazier response to this illness, but you didn't. Thanks for teaching me to persevere."

If patients have no awareness of positives, probe them about "exceptions" to their misery.

Even those with some appreciation of positives in their lives can benefit from creating a list of the gifts and graces of illness, or just of the good seconds they've recently experienced.

Avoid creating "pat" theological answers.

In an attempt to positively reframe a patient's concern, avoid trite answers. Such answers can cause harm. For example:

- "God needed him more" can be interpreted as "You didn't need him enough."

- "She's in a better place" can be translated as "You didn't make the world nice enough for her."

- "God does not give you more than you can carry" leaves the patient wishing he or she wasn't so strong![19]

EXERCISE 6.3

Positively reframe the following:

1. Neuropathic pain from cancer treatments.

_____

_____

2. "The nurses don't spend very much time in my room."

_____

_____

3. Blindness from diabetes mellitus.

_____

_____

4. "I have such a moon face! My whole body looks swollen."

_____

_____

See "Answers for Exercises," page 135.

Macro-skill 4: Religious practices

Religious practices (e.g., prayer, reading scripture, attending religious services) are related to good health outcomes.[20] These practices, of course, are chosen by the patient, and they intertwine with that patient's culture. Although religious practices cannot be imposed on patients, the HCP's role can be one of "cheerleading." That is, the HCP can affirm patients' use of helpful religious practices. For example, an anxious Buddhist patient can be reminded of his religious practice of meditation and how it can reduce anxiety. If appropriate, the HCP can also universalize a patient's religiousness by commenting on how others in similar situations have found meaning, courage, and strength from their religion.

Sometimes, it is healing to participate with the patient in a religious practice. Observing these guidelines can help HCPs to employ religious rituals with clients in ways that are ethical:

- First, try to understand the client's spiritual needs, resources, and preferences.

- Employ religious practices with permission; respect the client's expressed wishes.

- Do not prescribe or push religious beliefs or practices.

- Strive to understand your own spiritual beliefs and needs before addressing those of others.

- When it is appropriate to employ religious practices with patients, do so in a manner that is authentic and in harmony with your spiritual beliefs.[21]

Sometimes the patient requests that the HCP participate with him or her in a religious practice. At such times, consider the principles introduced in chapter five about self-disclosure. For example, after reading scripture to a patient, debrief by asking something such as, "What was going through your mind as I was reading?"

Ultimately, the goal of participating in religious practices with patients is to foster spiritual health. Although religion typically nurtures persons' spirituality, it can also "mask the face of God"[22] or hamper healthy spirituality. Refrain, therefore, from misusing religious practices in ways that block spiritual healing. For example, don't use religious rituals as a way to avoid exploration of uncomfortable spiritual suffering if exploration is needed. (See chapter seven, FAQs 5, 6, 7, 8, 10, and 11 for more information about addressing patient religiosity.)

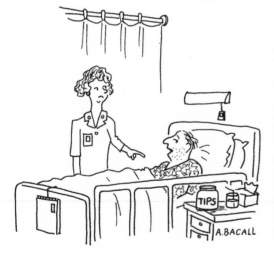

"That jar is not for money. It's for coping tips I can use to satisfy my spiritual needs."

Tips for praying with patients

Because prayer is an important religious practice in most religions of the world, most patients pray.[23] An HCP who prays with a patient is communicating to that patient that there is an ultimate power or resource; this allows hope. Patients occasionally ask HCPs, "Will you pray with me?" More likely, however, patients do not ask, but warmly welcome an HCP's sensitively worded offer to pray. A few suggestions about praying with patients, therefore, are offered here.[24]

- When asking patients if they would like you to pray with them, ask in a way that allows them to comfortably refuse. For example, "Often at times like this, people really want to pray with someone; would you like me to pray for you now?" Respect the answer.

- Consider the possible motivations prompting a patient's request for prayer. Patients who request prayer may want to test the HCP's attitudes or sincerity, to feel close to the HCP, to partake of the HCP's power, or to find spiritual comfort.

- Assess what kind of prayer the patient would like, as well as how he or she prefers to pray. While most Americans practice a conversational style of prayer, a patient may prefer other forms of prayer, such as meditational, ritual, or petitionary prayers.

- If the only type of prayer experience you and the patient feel comfortable with is a silent "thinking positive thoughts" in the presence of God and each other, your shared silence will be healing. Indeed, some would argue that prayer begins when words fail.

- Remember that prayer is encountering God with loving intention, and not the invocation of magic or manipulative preaching. Avoid praying in ways that either raise false hopes or block expression of innermost feelings.

- Conversational prayer is an opportunity to summarize the patient's feelings and experience. After listening to a patient's concerns, prayer that summarizes these concerns not only shows the patient you have listened, but also models that these concerns can be brought to God.

- Don't use prayer as an avoidance mechanism or as a substitute for relating. Although saying a prayer sometimes serves as an escape hatch from a painful topic or a pained patient, remember that prayer can be a springboard for deeper discussion.

- Even when they do not request a prayer, patients are often buoyed when a HCP simply—and sincerely—offers, "I'll be praying for you." Never feel you have to pray explicitly, because God is present regardless of the practice of any formal religion.

- Be alert to the fact that, for some, prayer brings spiritual doubts and distress to consciousness. For example, patients can be angry at God because they perceive their prayers have not been answered. This can raise questions about whether God is powerful or loving, or whether they are praying correctly. Healing is likely if this spiritual suffering is explored with the distressed patient rather than by blithely suggesting, "Pray more."

EXERCISE 6.4

Ann, a patient who is having difficulty talking about an emotional/spiritually painful topic, appears to disengage from conversing about it by asking you, "Will you pray for me?" What response would contribute to her healing?

_____

_____

_____

See "Answers for Exercises," page 136.

7 FAQs

This chapter discusses frequently asked questions (FAQs) and miscellaneous information essential to listening and responding to expressions of spiritual pain.

1. What do I do when a patient talks on and on and I have to go? What do I say to a patient when I need to leave and don't want to be rude?

Listen briefly, as time permits, and then summarize what he or she has said to you. Once you have summarized the message the patient gave you (i.e., you let him or her know that you really did hear and understand), tell him or her about your need to leave. For example, "You're disappointed about your family not visiting. I'd like to explore this more with you; however, I need to go."

Or you may need to redirect the patient if you need some information from them. For example, "I hear how frustrated you are about being here. I need to change the subject, however, and ask you about the medications you have been taking at home."

"Doorstep confessions" sometimes occur. You begin to leave the room and then the patient begins to disclose his or her spiritual pain. You can say something like, "That is a very important point. I can't address it now. Can you bring it up when . . . ?"

Someone who keeps talking is often someone who never feels

listened to. Show patience in your voice while firmly redirecting him or her or disengaging from him or her. Using phrases such as, "I'd like to hear more . . ." or "Perhaps we'll have time later to talk about this . . ." can soften the blow—if you are sincere.

2. Even when I do have a little time to listen, how do I deal with the patient who talks too much?

Patients who talk excessively are frustrating for many HCPs! HCPs may want to enjoy a two-way conversation that shows they care, or they may want to "get a word in edgewise" so that they can be therapeutic. If a patient talks too much, neither goal can be met.

An excessive talker is often a person with a need to be defensive.[1] Talking too much may indicate that the patient is afraid of talking about something or of becoming more self-aware. By talking too much, the patient keeps his or her helpers—and him- or herself, at a distance.

Try the following approach:

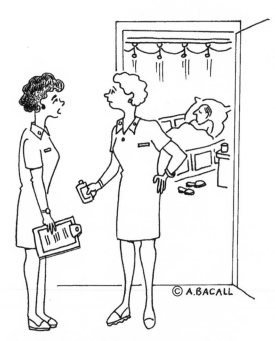

"We really should talk about how time constraints preclude applying the skills we were taught, to deal with spiritual distress, but I have to run."

- After letting the patient talk for five to ten minutes, interrupt with a statement like, "Forgive me for interrupting, but I won't be able help you think about this concern unless I can say a few things here and there. Let me see if I'm hearing you correctly now . . . " [offer a restatement or reflection that sums what the patient has said thus far]

- If the patient continues to talk too much, the HCP can subsequently interrupt (may need to hold up a hand even) and say something like, "Excuse me again, but I want to make sure I understand you. . . ."[2]

It is important to remember to keep your anger in check when you respond to excessive talkers.

3. What if the patient does not want to talk about his or her spirituality, but I know he or she would benefit from doing so?

Respect patient privacy. If a patient declines spiritual support, honor that wish. Ask yourself: Whose needs am I trying to meet? It may be that *you* have a need to provide solace to this patient, to correct his or her irrational religious beliefs, to make the patient experience spiritual realities the way you do.

It is also possible that this patient has adequate sources of spiritual support. Research has documented that nurses and physicians are not the first people patients look to for spiritual support.[3] Patients typically receive spiritual support from their family, friends, and personal clergy. A study of 224 cancer patients and family caregivers about what prerequisites they want to see in a nurse before receiving spiritual care indicated that genuine kindness and relationship (i.e., "Get to know me first") was more important than sharing similar beliefs or having training.[4]

If you have developed respect, rapport—relationship, then the patient may become interested in talking with you about spiritual matters. To show you care, you need to provide competent physical or technical care. When you expertly care for his or her cardiac condition, for example, the patient may then be receptive to spiritual care for his or her emotionally broken heart. If circumstances prevent you from developing a close relationship with a patient, remember what chaplains teach: "There's a lot of religion in a cup of cold water." That is, you give spiritual care even when you show compassion in common ways.

Also, remember that talking about what brings hope, what comforts, what is meaningful, and so forth, is talking about spirituality. Use the basic skills of chapter five. You can explore profound spiritual matters without ever using God language or religious terms.

4. How do I answer a patient who asks a "why" question?

"Why" questions come in many forms: Why me? Why not me? Why me instead of someone else? Why did it happen? (What caused it? What is to blame?) Why do bad things happen, especially to good people? Such questions are spiritually distressing, in part because they are unanswerable. Even the more temporal question of causation has a spiritual dimension because it has embedded in it the ultimate question of why does tragedy happen? And for those with a belief in God, fundamental questions are exposed: How can an all-powerful, loving God justify suffering?[5]

Several researchers have theorized and documented how many patients experience a spiritual transformation as a result of their suffering.[6] This transformation can manifest with:

- perceived changes in self (e.g., "I never knew until this how strong a person I am");

- a changed sense of relationships with others (e.g., "I am more sensitive towards others with similar suffering"); and

- a changed spirituality or philosophy of life (e.g., "Life seems more precious and now I do what is really important to me").

Some patients who ask "why," however, appear to get "stuck" in the abyss of asking an unanswerable question.[7] These patients are frustrated by the question, and sometimes appear depressed. Thus, an appropriate spiritual care goal for the patient asking "why?" is personal transformation.

While it is unwise to raise a "why" question for a patient, the patient who does ask such a question should be encouraged to give it voice. The techniques of chapter five will allow you to help the patient express the deeper meanings of asking "Why?" As with other deeply painful topics, the patient may be able to tolerate a limited amount of time discussing the topic. Follow the patient's cues, recognizing that the cognitive process of making sense of "why" involves approach as well as avoidance. Acknowledge for the patient that this is a struggle.

To support this process of transformation, you can ask open questions that hint at the potential benefits or positive meanings of suffering. For example:

- What has this experience taught you? (Or: What would you like to learn from this experience? What would it take to learn this?)

- What have you learned about yourself during this illness? (Or: What would you like to learn about yourself from this illness? What would it take to learn it?)

- How has this illness affected your attitude toward life?

- What are some of the good things that have resulted from this tragedy?

- It sounds like asking "why?" has not been helpful. Would it be more helpful to ask "wherefore?"

Be careful, however, never to impose positive interpretations on patients. Let patients lead you to where they find positive meaning. (See chapter six on resilience and reframing.)

5. How do I respond to someone with unhelpful spiritual beliefs?

Unhelpful spiritual beliefs are beliefs that, ultimately, prevent a patient from living fully. Unhelpful spiritual beliefs can be manifested by diminished hope, prolonged aimlessness, sarcasm, acting rigidly, self-centeredness, and a tendency to destroy relationships. Some research about negative religious coping links it with poor psychological adaptation to illness or caregiving.[8] For example, people who believe God is punishing or abandoning them, hold unresolved religious doubts and anger at God, and are in conflict about church dogma are more distressed than those who use positive religious coping. Thus, HCPs who can support patients to change their unhelpful religiosity into helpful religiosity are promoting spiritual and mental health.

How can the HCP respond? Here are some tips:

- Ask the patient in a sensitive manner if the beliefs you privately hold in question are helpful. For example:

  PT: "My husband is dying . . . I guess it's God's will."
  RN: "How comforting is that way of thinking?"

  Alternate queries could include: "What do you wish you could believe?" (And then: "What keeps you from believing this?") "How does this belief fit with your belief about [state helpful belief, e.g., your image of a loving God]"?

- Remember, to be nonthreatening, avoid starting any of these questions with the word "why."

- Encourage the patient to consult his or her spiritual leader, if appropriate. Sometimes the patient simply has "bad information."

Most patients will self-correct. Asking the patient to summarize his or her beliefs and/or asking one of the above questions will often stimulate a helpful restructuring. If not, recommend a referral to a spiritual care specialist such as a trained chaplain. Sometimes, the patient will ask you about your beliefs. Follow the self-disclosure guidelines in chapter five when responding.

Be careful, however, when you judge another's beliefs as unhelpful. Because the patient's beliefs are different from your own does not make them unhelpful. For example, a patient who says his or her loved one died because "it was God's will" may seem to you to be expressing unhelpful thinking. But it may be very comforting to the patient who trusts an all-powerful God uncritically.

The following story illustrates how "unhelpful" spiritual beliefs can be addressed in health care settings. Ruth, a forty-nine-year-old Christian Scientist, was pressured by her non–Christian Science family members to go to a hospital to have her pain checked. Various tests confirmed that Ruth had metastatic cancer. Specialists began to discuss the advanced extent of her disease with Ruth. She became overwhelmed with all the information and found the hospitalization was interfering with her spiritual practice of mind concentration. Consequently, she asked for no further information and said she wanted to leave the hospital so that she could reengage in the spiritual disciplines that gave her peace and comfort. The staff were distressed; Ruth was "in denial." Fortunately, an understanding physician discharged Ruth to an extended care facility that agreed to care for her while honoring her beliefs.

6. What if a patient tries to preach to me or prove his or her beliefs by showing me certain scriptural passages?

Remember that your goal with a patient is to help him or her understand the feelings and meanings within the illness experience so that he or she may have self-awareness. When a patient tries to prove some religious belief to you, respond in ways that allow the understanding of the feelings and meanings behind the preaching. For example, "I'm sensing that there is a lot hinging on this belief you're sharing," or, "What makes this doctrine so important to you?"

Sometimes patients will want to read a passage of their holy scripture to you, or they will tell you a story from it that shapes their thinking. For example, many patients find comfort from the biblical story of Job (whom God allows to endure intense suffering as he learns to remain in awe of the mystery and power of the Creator and Sustainer). A Swiss clergyman who dialogued with Sigmund Freud wrote, "Tell me what you find in the Bible, and I will tell you what you are."[9] Patients do tell HCPs much about themselves when they argue their beliefs or talk about religious stories.

7. What do I say to patients who believe a miracle will cure them of their disease?

Use the micro-skills introduced in chapter five to help these patients recognize the underlying need expressed by their desire for a "miracle" (e.g., a need to feel loved, a need to believe there is a trustable God). For example, you may respond with: "If I hear you correctly, your belief is that a cure would be the only way to know that God loves you." Such exploration may allow patients to reframe their definition of miracle. Rather than viewing the miracle as a cure, the miracle may be life itself or that loved ones are present to provide comfort.

Wanting God to rescue us by performing a miracle depicts a narrow image of God that does injustice to both the mysteries of God and to the human experience.[10] Patients can be encouraged to explore more encompassing views of God. For example: "Tell me more about how you think God works in people's lives." "I think I'm hearing conflicting viewpoints from you about how God is. One is that God is a rescuer, but another image sees God as a comforting friend during times of loss." Such exploration, however, will likely take time and more expertise. Make a referral.

8. What if a patient confesses guilt to me? What if it is an inappropriate guilt?

For many, healing occurs in the act of spoken confession to another. Because serious illness may bring to consciousness a sense of true guilt, HCPs sometimes become the receivers of confessed wrongs. If this occurs, inwardly recognize the sacredness of the act and allow the patient to explore the meaning of his or her guilt and the source of forgiveness. Such restitution is constructive, allowing healing within persons and relationships. If the patient is religious, suggest that he or she discuss this with clergy. As appropriate, use the techniques of chapter five to provide responses that will allow further inner exploration. For example: "My hunch is that you're really wanting to release the anger you've been carrying," or "What makes you want to say 'I'm sorry' to your friend now?" Or, "I'm guessing you might be wondering how other people find forgiveness" [and follow cues to determine appropriateness of self-disclosure].

Sometimes, however, patients will express a false or inappropriate guilt. This "guilt" is inwardly destructive: "Though it [false guilt] speaks with authority it develops phony people."[11] Statements from patients that may illustrate false guilt include: "I didn't think I could take care of mom and my family, but now that mom's gone I feel guilty because I should've kept her in my home," or "I shouldn't have done it, it shows I'm stupid . . . a failure." (Notice the use of "shoulds" and the confusion between shame and regret.) A response that may be helpful is: "I'm guessing you're feeling a bit guilty now. Do you think the guilt you have is the sort that will ultimately heal you or hurt you?" Whereas some patients with false, destructive guilt may gain the perspective they need from talking with you, they will probably need a referral to a mental or spiritual health care expert.

It is not unusual for patients to explain their illness or tragedy as punishment for past sins. While many diseases are outcomes of poor health habits (e.g., smoking, promiscuity), unresolved guilt is unhealthful. Patients can take the guilt they have about bad things they have done in the past, intensify it, and place it onto their illness. This displacement is even more likely if they do not get better and they feel they have disappointed those have tried to help them.[12] Carrying such guilt can provide some explanation for an otherwise unexplainable experience. That is, it is easier for some people to say, "I'm sick because I sinned," than to find another reason for their disease.

Patients with intense guilt may actually be reflecting inwardly an anger they hold towards another but are unable to recognize.[13] That is, people with lots of guilt may be indirectly saying they feel alienated from important people in their lives; their feeling bad gives a reason for why others have mistreated or neglected them. For these patients, it is easier to say, "I was treated badly because I was bad," rather than to accept that they were unjustly or capriciously treated. These complex spiritual problems are best referred to a spiritual or mental health professional.

9. How do I deal with a patient who is really angry?

Anger is energy created in response to a perceived threat. It can be directed outwardly or inwardly (depression). If the anger is being used to harm the self or others, introduce clear social and physical boundaries. Otherwise, you can use the basic skills in chapter five to help the patient become aware of his or her anger and to indirectly communicate that you are willing to be present even amidst the anger, if he or she wants that. An example of a response that reflects feelings is: "You are furious right now because you feel unheard."

Often patients will direct anger at those who are helping them. The root cause of the anger, however, can be the injustice of their victimization, the tragedy of their illness, the seeming abandonment of God, and other spiritual reasons. So that you do not respond defensively, remind yourself, "This is not about me." Instead, ask questions such as:

- What are you most angry about? (vs. "What are you *really* angry about?")

- How frustrated do you feel about . . . ? (Notice the diminutive form of the feeling of anger.)

- Have you ever felt this way before? How did you deal with it?

When a patient is able to be reflective about the anger:

- What do you think anger is? Is it bad? When you get angry, what do you do with that strong feeling? Can you think of some benefits you could gain from feeling angry? How might you direct this energy in a good way?

Remember that intense, current emotions are the hardest to talk about—harder than previous or less intense emotions. Recognize that you will need to approach the topic with tentativeness and sensitivity. Patients may deny initial observations you make about their feelings. Reword your observations to help them clarify their feelings (see chapter five).

10. I don't know all the different religious perspectives, so I'm afraid of saying something inappropriate. What do I do?

If you remain sensitive to this possibility, it is unlikely you will offend. When you begin discussing something that is likely to be affected by a patient's unique religious perspective, you might make a preface like, "I'm afraid of offending you because I don't know much about your religion. Can you let me know when I don't seem to understand you?" Or better, if time permits, ask an open question such as, "What should I know about your religious beliefs and practices?" or "How do your beliefs influence [topic of discussion]?"

Although you can read about health-related beliefs and practices of different world religions,[14] you may also learn from your patients who come from diverse religious backgrounds. Regardless of how much information you possess about religiosity, you cannot know how each patient will interpret or ascribe to a religion. Some Jews believe in a heaven, while others do not. Some Buddhists will pray to Buddha just as some Christians pray to God, while others do not. Variety in belief and practice exists not only between religions, but also among those of the same religious tradition. Sensitivity and use of the skills presented in chapter five can prevent embarrassment over not knowing a patient's unique religious perspective.

11. Are there any cultures or religions that think it is taboo to talk about spirituality with a HCP?

When approached with sensitivity and respect, especially in the context of a warm relationship, most patients will probably be appreciative of any inquiry you make about their spiritual health. There are no cultures or religions known to prohibit discussion of spiritual matters. Sometimes patients will prefer to discuss spiritual matters with someone of their own religion or philosophical orientation.

When discussing spiritual matters with some conservative or orthodox Jews, you may need to avoid using the terms "God" or "Jehovah." Some Jews consider these terms too holy for use in common conversation. You may want to ask, "In everyday conversation, what word do you use to describe that Higher Power?"

12. How can I talk with a patient about spiritual distress when I am not religious?

Remember, there is a difference between religion and spirituality. Regardless of your religiousness or lack thereof, you can implement the caring skills presented in chapter five. An HCP does not have to be religious to reflect feelings, ask open questions, and so forth.

Look for the spiritual common denominator between you and the patient. For example, you may both believe that love is one of the greatest virtues and that showing compassion for others is an ultimate purpose for which to live. Or, you may both accept there is some Ultimate Other or Sacred Source by which to orient one's life. Although you may have different labels and beliefs about this entity, you can begin to understand the patient's perspective and nurture spiritual awareness.

Although an institutionalized form of religion may not be nurturing to you right now, you inevitably have various spiritual beliefs and practices. You will bring your spirituality to the bedside. The HCP's religious biases for or against religion must be kept in check. Such biases cannot be kept in check, however, unless the HCP is aware of them. Understanding your own spirituality will help you to understand and respond to another's spiritual distress (see chapter two).

13. How can I support another's faith when my own is challenged or nonexistent?

You do not have to be perfect! Such an illusion, in fact, could be detrimental to accompanying others in their spiritual distress. Review chapter two to remember that *with* your woundedness you become a healer. Recognize, however, how your challenged or nonexistent "faith" could enter into your conversation with a patient and let it do so only for therapeutic purposes.

Consider an example that illustrates how an HCP with challenged or nonexistent faith can still provide spiritually healing responses to a patient:

PT, a victim of a disaster who has just lost a limb and a family member: "How could there be a loving God when this [expletive deleted] happens? For crying out loud . . . !"

HCP, wondering if there is a God or, if there is, if God could really be omnipotent and loving: "It is hard, it seems, to put trust in a God that exists while horrific stuff happens." Or, "Your whole body and soul is screaming out for a God that can be in control and be loving."

These responses name the deep spiritual pain and allow the victim to find perspective on his or her tragedy. These statements simply apply the skills presented in chapter five. How different these responses are from the following inappropriate self-disclosures: "I know. I've been asking the same thing"; "Yes, this just confirms my atheist beliefs. Erasing the idea of God gave me more mental health"; or, "But there is a God, you just have to have faith!"

14. When should I make a referral to a chaplain or other spiritual care expert?

The answer may seem obvious. When you don't have time, when you don't know what to say—when you can't help and you perceive that help is needed. In addition, you should call on spiritual and/or mental health care experts when a patient wants specialized theological knowledge or is living with a dangerous religiosity.

15. How do I broach the subject of spirituality with a patient?

The skills presented in this workbook assume that patients will introduce the subject. This workbook has also assumed that HCPs often fail to recognize the spiritual dimension inherent in many patients' comments and cries for help. The more tuned in you are, the more spirituality you will hear in others' conversations. The patient who says he is "bored looking at the ceiling 24/7" is describing a lack of fulfilling activity and stifled creativity, a thwarted sense of purpose. The burned-out colleague becomes a colleague searching for meaning in work or thirsting for respect. The friend, abandoned in childhood, who talks about her work to become a member of a club, becomes the friend who is talking about her search for belonging and a worthy identity—her need to be loved.

Whereas patients do bring spiritual issues into dialogue with HCPs, there may be times when the HCPs would like to steer the conversation toward a more overt discussion of spirituality. Variations on the question "What is helping you to cope with this illness/situation now?" usually will bring spiritual coping skills to light. Variations include questions such as: "What gives you the strength/hope you need now?" "What do you find most comforting in all of this?" "How are you dealing with this?" The assessment questions in FAQ 16 will also be useful.

16. How do I conduct a spiritual assessment?

Experts recommend a two-tiered approach to spiritual assessment:[15]

1. First, conduct a general, superficial assessment to ascertain spiritual beliefs and practices relevant to health care. This assessment can be completed with two questions: "What spiritual beliefs and practices would be important for your health care team to know?" "How would you like your health care team to nurture your spiritual health?" (This assessment meets the Joint Commission on Accreditation for Healthcare Organizations' requirement for spiritual assessment.)

2. Second, if there is evidence from the initial screening or subsequent observation suggesting spiritual or religious distress (or risk of it), then conduct a more in-depth assessment that focuses on the area of distress. For example, if a patient asks, "Why me?" then a spiritual assessment targeting how the patient ascribes meaning to life and to tragedy would provide information to guide therapeutics. For example, "Tell me more about what makes you ask this question." "Have you ever wondered it before? If so, how did you answer it before?" "What do you think will help you now to live with this question?"

This approach to spiritual assessment is appropriate considering the limited time and training of HCPs who are not spiritual care experts.

Long lists of spiritual assessment questions, however, are available elsewhere.[16] One excellent listing of questions includes:

- What sustains you through this illness?

- What gives you hope when coping with this illness is most difficult?

- Who truly understands what you are experiencing with this illness?

- How do you find comfort in your suffering? How do you find some moments of joy despite being ill?

- For what are you most deeply grateful?

- How does your life matter? What is your best sense as to what your life is about and how this illness fits in it?[17]

Remember that you can observe spiritual health through the behaviors of a patient. For example, is there anything in the patient's environment indicative of religious coping (e.g., prayer beads, religious cards, religious jewelry or clothing)? How do the patient's relationships with others (e.g., you, visitors, family) indicate spiritual health? What does the patient's mood and attitude indicate? And so forth.

17. How do I approach spiritual care with a difficult patient?

Illness, trauma, and other major life transitions sometimes contribute to regressive or difficult behavior such as passivity, preoccupation with past mistakes, whining, manipulating, and being belligerent. These behaviors actually show a stressed patient's yearning for someone to protect and nurture him or her.[18] Regressive behaviors have been described as being essentially a search for the "true self."[19] That is, serious illness takes away a person's identity and disrupts what is ordinary for that person. Because of this threat to adult identity, a patient's childhood fears and the accompanying regressive behaviors emerge. Your compassionate presence will allow difficult patients to regress, gather together their disparate pieces, and rebuild their identity and sense of self.[20]

18. Pretend I'm Christian and my patient is Wiccan or atheist. How do I help someone who practices a spirituality that is very different from mine?

Your care that supports patients' spiritual healing is not care that involves converting them to your way of thinking. Rather, through your responses to their expressions of suffering, you can help them to become more self-aware, more at ease with who (and for you, perhaps, whose) they are. Be respectful and avoid appearing shocked or antagonistic. Make a referral to a specialist if it is appropriate.

19. How can I apply the skills I've learned from this book to my work with children?

You can adapt and use these skills with children. As with adults, children describe their spiritual health and challenges through the stories they tell, behaviors, and so forth. And as with adults, they can learn spiritual principles from the stories that caregivers tell. As you create responses, consider the child's cognitive and faith development stage to determine what language will be age appropriate. Does he or she think concretely and literally about spiritual concepts like God and heaven? Or mythically and abstractly? Follow the child's cues about how to talk.

Children's spirituality reflects or interacts with that of their authority figure(s) (e.g., parents). The spiritual beliefs and practices of the authority figure(s) will be trusted and used by the child. Thus, many of the cues for how to talk with a child will come from that child's parents or guardian. Generally, it is not until the teenage years and young adulthood, when children can reason abstractly, that they begin to independently construct their own spiritual beliefs and practices.

Young children are especially honest and authentic. Mirroring this authenticity is vital to a healing relationship with a child. Perhaps, this authenticity led William Wordsworth to describe a child's spirituality in this way:

> Not in entire forgetfulness
> And not in utter nakedness,
> But trailing clouds of glory do we come
> From God, who is our home;

Heaven lies about us in our infancy!
Shades of the prison house begin to close
Upon the growing boy . . .[21]

Remembering Wordsworth's poetry about how as young children we are closer to God or more spiritually sensitive than we are as adults can help HCPs to respect a child's spiritual journey.

20. How can I apply the skills I've learned from this book to my work with persons with dementia?

The guidelines and tips for listening and responding to patients described here do apply to those with dementia as well. Know, however, that when interacting with those with dementia, you will not always be communicating on an intellectual level. The more the dementia has progressed, the less intellectual communication can occur. Therefore, focus more on listening and responding to the emotional and physical expressions. If, for example, a patient with advanced Alzheimer's disease speaking gibberish sounds frustrated, respond with a statement that recognizes that frustration. Although the patient will not cognitively understand, the tone of your voice and the look on your face that will accompany such a statement will likely be recognized at some level.

Remember that the disjointed phrases and stories persons with dementia speak offer a window to their world. Even if you cannot knit these pieces together for them, trying can help you to stay curious and engaged. For those with milder dementia, the strategies of promoting resilience and reframing are especially helpful.

21. I am okay with these workbook exercises, but it takes me a long time. How can I be ready to respond quickly when a patient expresses deep spiritual pain?

These skills require lots of practice! The curious and creative wounded healer, in fact, will always be "practicing." Remember, also, that it is respectful to take time to think carefully before responding.

8 Putting It All Together

Many specific details have been given in this workbook. You may be wondering how it all fits together. The exercises in this chapter will help you begin to integrate the various skills introduced in this workbook.

Let's practice!

EXERCISE 8.1

Analyze the following interaction between Chuck, skilled nursing facility resident, and his health care professional (HCP), a nurse:

RN1: Hi, Sweetie! How ya' doing this morning?

PT1: Oh, not so good, honey.

RN2: Why not? Today's the day that your son comes to visit. You always like that.

PT2: Yeah, but I didn't sleep so well last night. And the night nurses, they didn't answer me when I called. So I wet my bed, then had to lay in it for a long time. They're just so lazy, those night nurses.

RN3: I know it must seem that way, Chuck. I know they were really busy last night. I'm sure they didn't mean to ignore you. So have you gotten cleaned up now?

PT3: [with anger] Yeah, now I am. But I'm really upset when I can't pee in the bathroom. You know, it is just so . . .

RN4: Oh, I know. But thankfully, Chuck, it doesn't happen very often, right?

PT4: Yeah. But it is just so embarrassing when it does! You know, once I prayed to God that this wouldn't happen to me.

RN5: So, what are you and your son going to do today during his visit?

PT5: Well, hopefully, I won't pee in my pants!

RN6: [laughs] Good one, Chuck!

PT6: [unenthused] I suppose we'll just sit and watch TV together like we always do. He doesn't talk to me much.

RN7: So, when is he coming? I forgot, where does he live?

PT7: 10:30 a.m. He lives just across town.

RN8: Well, I know what you can do. You can just start asking him questions. Like what his kids are up to. How his work is. Maybe if you ask him questions, he'll ask you some, too. Then you can actually have a two-way conversation for a change. I know I had to work hard at doing this with my mother, and it worked pretty well. Now she tells me about everyone she's talked to, what she sees on TV, and stuff like that. I think you'll feel better if you try this approach.

PT7: Maybe so.

RN8: Well, I'd better get going.

PT8: Okay.

RN9: Bye Chuck.

PT9: Bye.

Review the "silencing responses" of chapter two, Exercise 2.4. Which ones do you observe here? Indicate with the appropriate number where in the above verbatim you observed the following:

☐ A. Changing the subject

☐ B. Inserting humor

☐ C. Giving a pat answer

☐ D. Imposing positivity

☐ E. Minimizing discomfort

☐ F. Imposing a solution, preaching

☐ G. Focusing on an unnecessary tangent

What are Chuck's biggest concerns?

_____

_____

What spiritual needs might underlie these concerns?

_____

_____

How would you respond to Chuck to help him become more spiritually aware? Write a response to replace RN5 that reflects Chuck's deeper feelings and their meaning.

_____

_____

EXERCISE 8.2

Tessa, seventy-two-year-old mother of Ron, is a home hospice patient. Analyze the following interaction.

HCP1: How are you feeling today?

PT1: Not very good. [looks depressed]

HCP2: It isn't that bad, is it?

PT2: This morning when I woke up, I was asking myself, "When is it going to end?" [long pause] Why is it so hard to die? [eyes getting red]

HCP3: I'm sorry, Tessa. [deep breath]

PT3: Because of my sickness, people around me are suffering. And that drives me nuts! [tears begin to roll]

HCP4: Why do you think that they are suffering?

PT4: Like Ron, he used to exercise in the morning. But now, because of me, he doesn't have time to do things that he likes to do anymore. I feel guilty. [sobbing, catching breath] The other day I got urine on my dress. I tried to change the dress myself. But I ended up making more mess. And Ron had to clean it up.

HCP5: Oh, come here, Tessa! [gives hug, rubs back]

PT5: Lord, have mercy. Just let me die. [sobbing]

HCP6: Wanting to take care of you is Ron's choice. Right now, taking care of you is his priority because he loves you very much. There is nothing that you need to feel guilty about. [hug again]

PT6: Maybe. [said unconvincingly]

HCP7: So, are the pain pills still working well enough?

Questions to prompt analysis:

Which silencing responses does the HCP use?

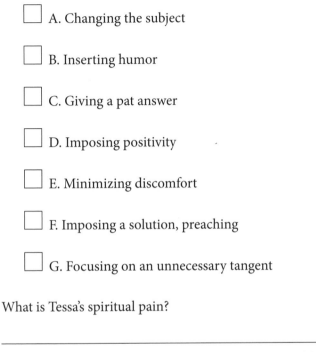

☐ A. Changing the subject

☐ B. Inserting humor

☐ C. Giving a pat answer

☐ D. Imposing positivity

☐ E. Minimizing discomfort

☐ F. Imposing a solution, preaching

☐ G. Focusing on an unnecessary tangent

What is Tessa's spiritual pain?

_____

Write two verbal responses to replace HCP6 that would be helpful:

1. _____

_____

2. _____

_____

EXERCISE 8.3

Brett, thirty-eight, is a person with AIDS and is in a transitional care unit. Analyze the following exchange.

HCP1: I hear you'll be leaving soon.

PT1: Yeah, I'm so glad to get out of here. I'm thirty-eight and living here with ninety-year-olds. That's just not right.

HCP2: How does that make you feel?

PT2: Depressed. People are dying around me. It's already bad enough that I am dying. I don't need to be reminded of death every second of every day. [PT appears angry.]

HCP3: You seem angry.

PT3: I am. Because it's taken me a long time to get out of here. I didn't mean to yell at you. I'm sorry. [PT looks away.]

HCP4: It's okay. Things have been difficult for you. I'm here, though, if there's anything you would like to talk about.

PT4: I don't understand what is expected from me. I just try to do things right, but they end up going wrong. Just when I think things can't get any worse, they do. [lights a cigarette] You know what's so funny? [smiles ironically] Some people try to convince me to stop smoking, when smoking is the least of my problems. It helps calm me down.

HCP5: [smiling back] Whose expectations?

PT5: Life's. God's. I don't know. You know how they say, "Do good and you will be rewarded?" Well, it's not true. [pause] Well, maybe I'm being punished for being a homosexual. My mother disowned me because of that. I thought I was in a monogamous relationship. I was faithful to Kevin. Not only did he break my heart, he gave me this disease. [starts to cry silently]

HCP6: [moves closer, places hand on Brett's arm]

PT6: [breathes deeply] I had finally come to terms with my condition. Just when I learned to deal with it, now I have this brain disease. Like having AIDS is not enough. Now I can't even move the left side of my body. [wipes tears away] I'm only thirty-eight. What did I do that was so wrong? Why me?

HCP7: [handing him a tissue] I don't know. [starts to tear up]

PT7: Thank you for listening. I know you didn't have to stay this long. [smiles and makes eye contact]

Questions to prompt analysis:

Which one of the following best describes Brett's spiritual pain?

  a) unabated physical pain
  b) betrayal or broken trust
  c) loss of dignity
  d) loss of purpose

What did this HCP do or say that promoted healing?

_____

_____

What could have been more effective?

_____

_____

See analyses for Exercises 8.1, 8.2, and 8.3 in "Answers for Exercises," pages 136–138.

EXERCISE 8.4

This exercise can be repeated each time you have a conversation with someone that you sense you were not as effective as you could have been to support healing.

Write down verbatim conversation(s) you had with a patient where a spiritual concern was raised, overtly or covertly. To maintain this patient's anonymity, use a pseudonym for the name. You may want to use the interaction you identified in chapter one, Exercise 1.1. Use the following questions to analyze your responses.

Did you . . .

☐ Listen with your head, heart, and muscles (i.e., intellect, feelings, body)?

☐ Understand what was said nonverbally?

☐ Let the patient do most of the talking?

☐ Change or avoid an uncomfortable subject?

☐ Give a pat answer?

☐ Impose positivity?

☐ Minimize discomfort

☐ Impose a solution, preach?

☐ Focus on an unnecessary tangent?

☐ Ask unnecessary questions?

☐ Interrupt helpful silence?

☐ Control the conversation (e.g., with lots of questions)?

☐ Use self-disclosure only after assessing if and why the patient wanted to hear your perspective?

☐ Vary the way you asked questions or made reflections?

☐ Ascertain the core theme?

☐ Address the deeper feeling(s) and their meaning?

☐ Keep your responses focused on the patient? In the present?

☐ Find that your responses encouraged the patient to explore further his or her issue or gain self-awareness?

What would you say differently, given another chance?

An encouraging word

This workbook provides techniques for how to talk with patients in ways that help them to gain awareness of their spirituality. Although practicing these techniques will allow you to be more comfortable and capable, it may feel daunting to implement them. Remember that who you are as a person and your sincere interest in the patient as a person are what matter most. Your compassion can often compensate for your imperfect talking technique. There is a Power greater than yourself, after all, that does the healing.

Answers for Exercises

Note: Your answers to patient scenarios will not be the same as those provided here. Please remember these are just some of the many possible responses.

Chapter 3

Exercise 3.5

RN2: The patient has just alluded to a lonely life. His deeper feelings may include feeling betrayed or abandoned by his children, estrangement from church, and an overall sense of isolation or loneliness. The nurse does not respond in a way that shows this suffering was heard. Although the patient may be experiencing such spiritual suffering, the nurse picks up on the overt religious behavior only.

The nurse asks an open-ended question. "Why" questions, however, can be threatening or judgmental—as this one could easily be interpreted. The PT2 response of avoiding the question suggests that the real answer is painful to discuss.

RN3: The nurse is focused on a minor detail that is insignificant given the deeper issue.

RN4: The nurse is eager to "push church!" A more fruitful query might be, "Tell me about how your past church experiences affect the way you relate to people at church now." In the PT4 response, the patient appears to be sidestepping.

RN5: Another tangential, irrelevant detail is asked.

RN6: This judgmental response clearly helps the patient to close an emotional door completely. The patient's response is to change the subject, another indicator of not being heard.

RN7: The nurse appears not to have heard the patient's earlier comments indicating that there is a problem with connecting to persons at church. The patients' verbal and nonverbal responses are indicators that the nurse's talk was not helpful; the patient probably just wants to get the nurse out of the room. (We do not know the problem. It could be that since becoming confined to a wheelchair, he is unable to attend, and because he does not want to be indebted to church members, he decides not to ask them for help. Or, it could be that the patient was offended by someone at church and feels estranged or angry. Or, the patient may feel angry at God and therefore wants to disassociate from any reminders of God.)

Conclusion

The RN's goal cannot be to fix the patient's spiritual problem. Rather, the RN is to listen and respond with care that allows the patient to process his own feelings and make decisions.

Chapter 4

Exercise 4.1

Appropriate answers:

1. This father is reevaluating his religious beliefs, his view of God—indicating not only his primal need for experiencing transcendence, but also for trustfully relating to God. He is also restructuring a worldview so that it continues to be meaningful.

2. This quadriplegic is trying to find meaning, to make sense of why this tragedy happened. She is also wondering what purpose—vocation, mission, calling—there is for her now.

3. This cancer survivor is jubilant and has a need to express this joy, as she needs to experience herself fully and authentically.

Exercise 4.2

Answers: 1. A, 2. B, 3. B, 4. A

Exercise 4.3

Commentary:

1. Quite safe. Although this PT does not have sophisticated language for explaining his religious beliefs, he is courageous enough—or desperate enough—to introduce the topic to his HCP. And he reintroduces it after the HCP digresses (HCP2/PT2). He does not shy away from this uncomfortable topic and is fairly receptive to letting the HCP explore it with him.

2. He balances concrete and abstract thinking about his spiritual pain.

3. PT8 indicates he is receptive to thinking in a new way about his spiritual pain and resources.

4. He uses religious idioms of "just praying and hoping," "penalized for sins," "just as soon go up there than down there," and "man upstairs."

5. The HCP identifies an incongruity in HCP8. Another incongruity is that he asks "why" in PT4, after stating an explanation in PT3. Clearly, the answer to "why" in PT3 is discomforting, so he continues to ask in PT4.

6. The PT's religion provides a negative meaning for the pain, and demonstrates an insecure attachment to God.

7. The HCP does a good job of restating and asking open questions. Use of these micro-skills does allow the PT to explore and gain insight (PT8). The HCP is skillful at not "taking the rug [of unhelpful religion] out from under his feet." Rather, the HCP en-

courages the patient to hear himself, to rethink and respond to his real issues. The patient probably needs a spiritual therapeutic that allows him to confess his sins. The HCP could have made a referral to clergy or to a spiritual care expert for this confession.

Chapter 5

Exercise 5.2

HCP1: Guidelines 1, 2, 4, 5, 9, and 11 were not followed. The HCP appears to have missed the real spiritual suffering that is occurring: Wondering *why I,* in particular, got this disease. Such patients sometimes wonder if there is a reason, if the disease is a punishment, or if they were selected because they were "strong enough." Instead of addressing this spiritual question, the HCP provides scientific information about the cause of the disease. While this may be appropriate at some point in this conversation, the explanation may be falling on unready ears—ears preoccupied by a painful spiritual question.

HCP2: At least 5, 6, and 11 were not followed. Possibly 3 and 4 also were not followed. This PT is talking intellectually about something that probably contributes to a spiritual struggle about being valuable, worthy, loved. Given his story (i.e., probably his childhood environment did not allow him to explore his inner feelings much) and his present "head" talk, he is unlikely to be helped by this HCP's feeling-oriented response.

HCP3: Guidelines 1, 2, 6, 7, 9, and 10 were not followed. Whereas the PT used "God," the HCP assumed with the patient meant "Jesus." Whereas the PT's sensory orientation was visual, the HCP's was auditory.

Exercise 5.3

Possible answer: Enter slowly [matching voice speed], speak calmly—yet maintain confidence, curl up your torso somewhat as you sit in the chair next to her bed, which you pull to allow you a 90–180 degree angle while being with her. You say, "I'm _____, and I'm so sorry to hear about the diagnosis. Allow long pause for her to respond. If she does not, "What are you thinking?" (Do not project what you think or feel she is thinking or feeling.) Accept whatever she says, and follow her cues. Do not be pushy for more information than she chooses to divulge now.

Exercise 5.4

Possible responses:

1. You're thinking, perhaps, it's impossible to right the wrong of hurting your wife.

2. Maybe the MS is leading you to conclude that you are unlovable, unsexy.

3. It seems like you're finding it hard to have any purpose for living when you are so dependent on others.

Exercise 5.5

Possible responses:

1. What's the hardest part to forgiving yourself?

2. Tell me about what you think love is. How might it be possible to make love again? (Or, What would it take to be wanted again?)

3. What's it like to be so dependent on others? (Or, What purpose might there be for you're being alive now?)

Exercise 5.7

Possible responses:

Single word: "You feel abandoned."

Phrase: "It makes you angry."

Experiential statement: "You feel God shouldn't let this happen." "You feel like you're dying on a cross, too."

Behavioral statement: "You feel ready for a fistfight with God."

Exercise 5.8

1–b, 2–c, 3–a, 4/5–d

Exercise 5.9

Case 1

Possible responses:

Basic: "It seems you're feeling pretty sure God will not heal you.

Advanced: "I'm wondering if maybe you're rather disappointed or angry that God isn't healing you."

Case 2

Possible responses:

Basic: "You're afraid of him dying."

Advanced: "Perhaps it is so scary to think about life without him that you don't let yourself think it is possible."

Chapter 6

Exercise 6.1

Case 1

Possible responses, after ascertaining that all physical care for her complaint has been provided: "Your story makes sense to me. You feel like you're a victim of poor nursing care, and maybe even a victim of a body that's wearing out." Or, "Your story about what happened makes me wonder if you're feeling helpless and if that's maybe making you afraid" [reflections of deeper feeling that connect story to the present]. "Have you ever felt like this before? How did you cope with it then?" [open questions to find resiliency]. "This story about falling; how do you think it might tell about other ways that you feel like you're falling down?" [open question that tries to integrate this episode into the larger picture of her life].

Case 2

Possible responses: "Interesting, Ken, it's like Tom's story is your story—bad luck, caprice. I'm wondering if that's been a theme in your life. What do you think?" Or, "How would you say that your life story matches Tom's?" "How did you make sense of the un-luckiness of Tom's death? . . . Is that how you want to make sense of your misfortune?"

Exercise 6.2

Possible response: "I'd like to suggest some questions that will take a minute to ponder. Maybe you'd like to write in your journal about them later. Just get comfy and let your body speak to you as you think about the answers. What is it about this situation that makes this ball heavy in your stomach? What word/idea makes you aware of the ball in your stomach? What is it that makes the ball heavy? Perhaps you could ask this heavy ball what it needs. What does it want to tell you?"

Exercise 6.3

Possible answers:

1. The pain reminds a person that he or she is very much alive.

2. The patient would have to be a lot sicker for the nurses to spend more time, or the patient has more time to spend in uninterrupted, quiet meditation.

3. Blindness is an opportunity to develop other senses more— to experience the world and life in a new way.

4. An altered body image forces exploration of what really makes one valuable—and it isn't looks.

Exercise 6.4

Possible response: "Sure, Ann, for what would you like me to pray?" Her answer will provide rich data; pray naming her deepest feeling(s), then note nonverbal communication to evaluate appropriateness of the prayer, or ask: "How was it for you, praying like this?" Often after praying with a patient, a silent presence is the best response—with a hug or hand squeeze, if appropriate.

Chapter 8

Exercise 8.1

A–RN3, 5
B–RN6
C–RN3
D–RN2, 4
E–RN4
F–RN8
G–RN7

What are Chuck's biggest concerns? urinary incontinence, relationship with son

What spiritual needs might underlie these concerns? Incontinence may threaten his sense of dignity and expose a loss of control over his body, all of which could weaken his self-worth. He also implies he may be disappointed about God not answering a prayer. His poor communication with his son may undermine his need to give and receive love, leave a legacy, and so forth.

How would you respond to Chuck to help him become more spiritually aware? Write a response to replace RN5. "It's humiliating to not be able to control your own body. And I'm wondering, too, if you might not only be frustrated at the nurses for letting this happen, but maybe also at God." This is just a possible answer.

Exercise 8.2

Analysis: Tessa is desperate to unload some of her spiritual pain, even though it is very difficult for her HCP to hear it. The HCP uses silencing responses of minimizing (HCP2), imposing positivity (HCP6), and changing the topic (HCP7). In HCP4, an intimidating "why" question is asked instead of a "how" or a "what" question. The HCP never allows Tessa to explore her deepest feelings; hence, spiritual healing is not fostered. The crux of Tessa's spiritual pain involves her desire to die because it is difficult to find meaning or purpose in being dependent on a child for even basic hygienic care. Healing responses could include: "I'm sensing that your eagerness to die is because you don't want to be a burden to your family." "Maybe being dependent on others makes you wonder if there is any purpose in staying alive." "If I hear you right, what's hard about dying is feeling like you're disrupting your family's life." "Tessa, what sorts of positives have come from having your son help you?" "Tell me a story about when you cared for one of Ron's messes. . . . How might your son's caring for your basic needs bring closure to all the caring you've given him throughout his life?"

Exercise 8.3

Analysis: Although Brett may have been struggling with all of these pains, b) broken trust is what he talks most about in this passage.

What did this health care professional do or say that promoted healing? This HCP clearly was perceived by Brett as compassionate. In spite of some less than perfect responses, Brett was able to explore or share his spiritual pain. The HCP did allow Brett to explore his feelings, although their meanings were not unpacked. The HCP refrains from offering any pat answers and avoiding his discomforting "why" question." The HCP was authentic in responding with "I don't know," but it may have caused Brett to discontinue the exploration.

What could have been more effective? The crux of Brett's spiritual pain lies in betrayal or broken trust. Life, his body, God, mother, and lover have all betrayed him. Some people are even trying to get him to stop smoking. They don't understand his more important problems, so how can they be trusted? From this sense of betrayal comes "why?" questions and a yearning for relationship—with people who won't leave him for death, too. He wonders what he did to earn these betrayals. Given these spiritual pains, responses such as the following would be more effective: [at HCP7] "Tell me if I'm off here, but it seems that you're really angry about being betrayed, betrayed by your body, your lover, your mom, your God, life. And now you're wondering if you did something to make these betrayals happen." Brett can then refine and further explore his deeper feeling. When appropriate, open questions exploring the meaning of his spiritual pain could be asked. For example, "You asked if there was something you did that was wrong. What do you think?" Or, "How did these betrayals to make you the person you are?" Or, "How does this betrayal feel in your body? . . . What does it look like? Where is it? . . . If this _____ could speak, what would it say to you?"

Notes

Chapter 1: Let's Begin!

1. J. W. Pennebaker, *Opening Up: The Healing Power of Expressing Emotions* (New York: Guilford, 1997); J. O. Greene and B. R. Burleson, eds., *Handbook of Communication and Social Interaction Skills* (Mahwah, NJ: Lawrence Erlbaum, 2003).

2. H. G. Koenig and H. J. Cohen, eds., *The Link between Religion and Health: Psychoneuroimmunology and the Faith Factor* (New York: Oxford University Press, 2002); J. S. Levin, *God, Faith and Health: Exploring the Spirituality-Healing Connection* (New York: John Wiley, 2001); D. A. Matthews, M. E. McCullough, D. B. Larson, H. G. Koenig, J. P. Swyers, and M. G. Milano, "Religious Commitment and Health Status: A Review of the Research and Implications for Family Medicine," *Archives of Family Medicine* 7, no. 2 (1998): 118–24.

3. "Charmides," in *The Dialogues of Plato*, trans. B. Jowett (New York: Random House, 1937), I.6.

4. D. Baldacchino and P. Draper, "Spiritual Coping Strategies: A Review of the Nursing Research Literature," *Journal of Advanced Nursing* 34 (2001): 833–41; H. G. Koenig, K. I. Pargament, and J. Nielsen, "Religious Coping and Health Status in Medically Ill Hospitalized Older Adults," *Journal of Nervous and Mental Disease* 186 (1998): 513–21; K. I. Pargament, *The Psychology of Religion and Coping* (New York: Guilford, 1997), 8; E. J. Taylor, "Spiritual Complementary Therapies in Cancer Care," *Seminars in Oncology Nursing* 21, no. 3 (2005): 159–63.

5. T. Bauer and C. R. Barron, "Nursing Interventions for Spiritual Care: Preferences of the Community-based Elderly," *Journal of Holistic Nursing* 13 (1995): 268–79; A. Hart Jr., R. J. Kohlwes, R. Deyo, L. A. Rhodes, and D. J. Bowen, "Hospice Patients' Attitudes Regarding Spiritual Discussions with Their Doctors," *American Journal of Hospice and Palliative Care* 20 (2003): 135–39; R. S. Hebert, M. W. Jenkes, D. E. Ford, D. R. O'Connor, and L. A. Cooper, "Patient Perspectives on Spirituality and the Patient-Physician Relationship," *Journal of General Internal Medicine* 16 (2001): 685–92; C. D. MacLean, B. Susi, N. Phifer, L. Schultz, D. Bynam, M. Franco, et al., "Patient Preference for Physician Discussion and Practice of Spirituality," *Journal of General Internal Medicine* 18 (2003): 38–43; G. McCord, V. J. Gilchrist, S. D. Grossman, B. D. King, K. E. McCormick, A. M. Oprandi, et al., "Discussing Spirituality with Patients: A Rational and Ethical Approach," *Annals of Family Medicine* 2 (2004): 356–61; E. J. Taylor and I. Mamier, "Spiritual Care Nursing: What Cancer Patients and Family Caregivers Want," *Journal of Advanced Nursing* 49, no. 3 (2005): 260–67.

6. J. A. Sanford, *Between People: Communicating One-to-One* (Ramsey, NJ: Paulist Press, 1982).

7. Pargament, *The Psychology of Religion and Coping*.

8. J. Luckmann, *Transcultural Communication in Nursing* (Albany, NY: Delmar, 1999).

9. M. A. Burkhardt and M. G. Nagai-Jacobson, *Spirituality: Living Our Connectedness* (Albany, NY: Delmar, 2002); E. J. Taylor, *Spiritual Care: Nursing Research, Theory, and Practice* (Upper Saddle River, NJ: Prentice Hall, 2002); H. G. Koenig, *Spirituality in Patient Care: Why, How, When, and What* (Philadelphia: Templeton Foundation Press, 2002).

10. Taylor, *Spiritual Care.*

11. H. J. Clinebell Jr., *Basic Types of Pastoral Counseling* (Nashville: Abington, 1966).

12. A. P. Dominic, "A Natural Principle of Spirituality," *Review for Religious* (September–October, 1988): 748–54.

13. Sanford, *Between People.*

14. W. West, *Psychotherapy and Spirituality* (London: Sage, 2000).

15. G. G. May, *Care of Mind: Care of Spirit: Psychiatric Dimensions of Spiritual Direction* (San Francisco: Harper & Row, 1982), 93.

16. M. Friedman, *The Healing Dialogue in Psychotherapy* (New York: Aronson, 1985).

Chapter 2: Preparing the Healer

1. Quote attributed to Knight, 1986, in C. R. Figley, ed., *Treating Compassion Fatigue* (New York: Brunner-Routledge, 2002).

2. H. J. M. Nouwen, *The Wounded Healer* (Garden City, NJ: Image Books, 1979), 72.

3. J. Stairs, *Listening for the Soul: Pastoral Care and Spiritual Direction* (Minneapolis: Fortress, 2000).

4. D. Parker, "Devils of Mercy," *Working Nurse*, July 18, 2005, 31, italics added.

5. T. Hora, *Beyond the Dream: Awakening to Reality,* 2nd ed. (New York: Crossroads, 1996), 79.

6. J. A. Sanford, *Between People: Communicating One-to-One* (Ramsey, NJ: Paulist Press, 1982).

7. J. L. Griffith and M. E. Griffith, *Encountering the Sacred in Psychotherapy* (New York: Guilford, 2002).

8. W. N. Grosch and D. C. Olsen, *When Helping Starts to Hurt: A New Look at Burnout Among Psychotherapists* (New York: Norton, 1994), 4.

9. A. M. Pines and E. Aronson, *Burnout: Causes and Cures*, 2nd ed. (New York: Free Press, 1988).

10. Grosch and Olsen, *When Helping Starts to Hurt.*

11. A. B. Baranowsky, "The Silencing Response in Clinical Practice: On the Road to Dialogue," in C. R. Figley, ed., *Treating Compassion Fatigue* (New York: Brunner-Routledge, 2002).

12. D. G. Larson, *The Helper's Journey: Working with People Facing Grief, Loss, and Life-Threatening Illness* (Champaign, IL: Research Press, 1993).

13. Baranowsky, "The Silencing Response in Clinical Practice."

14. V. Satir, *Of Rocks and Flowers*, video of Virginia Satir (Kansas City: Golden Triad Films, 1985).

Chapter 3: Listening: Beginning the Healing Response

1. L. A. Burton, "The Medical Patient: Compassionate Listening and Spirit-Mind-Body Care of Medical Patients," in R. B. Gilbert, ed., *Health Care and Spirituality: Listening, Assessing, Caring* (Amityville, NY: Baywood, 2002), 164.

2. J. Stairs, *Listening for the Soul: Pastoral Care and Spiritual Direction* (Minneapolis: Fortress, 2000), 34.

3. H. J. Clinebell Jr., *Basic Types of Pastoral Counseling* (Nashville: Abington, 1966).

4. J. A. Sanford, *Between People: Communicating One-to-One* (Ramsey, NJ: Paulist Press, 1982).

5. National Listening Association, http://www.listen.org, accessed October 2005.

6. J. Rowan, "Holistic Listening," *Journal of Humanistic Psychology* 26, no. 1 (1986): 83–102; P. Osterman and D. Schwartz-Barcott, "Presence: Four Ways of Being There," *Nursing Forum* 31, no. 2 (1996): 23–30.

7. Stairs, *Listening for the Soul*, 17.

8. M. Fowler and B. S. Peterson, "Spiritual Themes in Clinical Pastoral Education," *Journal of Training and Supervision in Ministry* 18 (1997): 46–54.

9. Clinebell, *Basic Types of Pastoral Counseling*.

10. J. L. Griffith and M. E. Griffith, *Encountering the Sacred in Psychotherapy* (New York: Guilford, 2002).

11. R. Dilts, *Applications of Neuro-Linguistic Programming* (Cupertino, CA: Meta, 1983).

12. Clinebell, *Basic Types of Pastoral Counseling*; Dilts, *Applications of Neuro-Linguistic Programming*; R. Dayringer, *The Heart of Pastoral Counseling: Healing through Relationship*, rev. ed. (New York: Haworth Pastoral Press, 1998); R. J. Lovinger, "Religious Issues," in *The Counseling Sourcebook: A Practical Reference on Contemporary Issues*, ed. J. L. Ronch, W. Van Ornum, and N. C. Stilwell (New York: Crossroad, 1994), 202–22.

13. W. R. Miller and S. Rollnick, *Motivational Interviewing: Preparing People for Change,* 2nd ed. (New York: Guilford, 2002).

14. Dayringer, *The Heart of Pastoral Counseling.*

15. Griffith and Griffith, *Encountering the Sacred in Psychotherapy.*

16. Dayringer, *The Heart of Pastoral Counseling.*

17. Sanford, *Between People.*

18. Lovinger, "Religious Issues."

19. Dayringer, *The Heart of Pastoral Counseling*; B. Rybarczyk and A. Bellg, *Listening to Life Stories* (New York: Springer, 1997).

20. Clinebell, *Basic Types of Pastoral Counseling.*

21. C. E. Hill and K. M. O'Brien, eds., *Helping Skills: Facilitating Exploration, Insight, and Action* (Washington, DC: American Psychological Association, 1999).

22. Sanford, *Between People.*

23. H. Brody, *Stories of Sickness* (New Haven: Yale University, 1987).

24. G. Egan, *The Skilled Helper: A Problem-Management and Opportunity-Development Approach to Helping,* 7th ed. (Pacific Grove, CA: Brooks/Cole, 2002).

25. Sanford, *Between People.*

Chapter 4: Making Sense of What You Hear

1. E. J. Taylor, *Spiritual Care: Nursing Research, Theory, and Practice* (Upper Saddle River, NJ: Prentice Hall, 2002).

2. H. J. Clinebell Jr., *Basic Types of Pastoral Counseling* (Nashville: Abington, 1966), 251.

3. J. L. Griffith and M. E. Griffith, *Encountering the Sacred in Psychotherapy* (New York: Guilford, 2002).

4. Clinebell, *Basic Types of Pastoral Counseling*; Griffith and Griffith, *Encountering the Sacred in Psychotherapy*; R. Dayringer, *The Heart of Pastoral Counseling: Healing through Relationship,* rev. ed. (New York: Haworth Pastoral Press, 1998); R. J. Lovinger, "Religious Issues," in *The Counseling Sourcebook: A Practical Reference on Contemporary Issues,* ed. J. L. Ronch, W. Van Ornum, and N. C. Stilwell (New York: Crossroad, 1994), 202–22; J. S. Savage, *Listening and Caring Skills in Ministry: A Guide for Pastors, Counselors, and Small Groups* (Nashville: Abington, 1996).

5. Griffith and Griffith, *Encountering the Sacred in Psychotherapy.*

6. Clinebell, *Basic Types of Pastoral Counseling*; Dayringer, *The Heart of Pastoral Counseling*.

7. R. J. Lovinger, "Religious Issues," in *The Counseling Sourcebook: A Practical Reference on Contemporary Issues*, ed. J. L. Ronch, W. Van Ornum, and N. C. Stilwell (New York: Crossroad, 1994), 202–22.

8. Dayringer, *The Heart of Pastoral Counseling*.

9. J. B. Ashbrook, *Minding the Soul: Pastoral Counseling as Remembering* (Minneapolis: Fortress, 1996).

10. J. W. Fowler, *Stages of Faith Development: The Psychology of Human Development and the Quest for Meaning* (San Francisco: Harper & Row, 1981).

11. Lovinger, "Religious Issues."

12. Ibid.

13. O. Pfister, quoted in Dayringer, *The Heart of Pastoral Counseling*, 53.

14. Griffith and Griffith, *Encountering the Sacred in Psychotherapy*.

15. Clinebell, *Basic Types of Pastoral Counseling*, 250.

16. K. I. Pargament, *The Psychology of Religion and Coping* (New York: Guilford, 1997); B. Cole, E. Benore, and K. Pargament, "Spirituality and Coping with Trauma," in *Spirituality, Health, and Wholeness: An Introductory Guide for Health Care Professionals*, ed. S. Sirajjakool and H. Lamberton (New York: Haworth Press, 2004), 49–76.

Chapter 5: Verbal Responses to Spiritual Distress: The Micro-skills

1. R. R. Carkhuff, *The Art of Helping*, 5th ed. (Amherst, MA: Human Resource Development Press, 1983); G. Egan, *Exercises in Helping Skills: A Manual to Accompany the Skilled Helper*, 6th ed. (Pacific Grove, CA: Brooks/Cole, 1998); C. E. Hill and K. M. O'Brien, eds., *Helping Skills: Facilitating Exploration, Insight, and Action* (Washington, DC: American Psychological Association, 1999); G. Goodman and G. Esterly, *The Talk Book* (Emmaus, PA: Rodale, 1988); O. C. Hammond, D. H. Hepworth, and V. G. Smith, *Improving Therapeutic Communication* (San Francisco,

CA: Jossey-Bass, 1977); D. G. Larson, *The Helper's Journey: Working with People Facing Grief, Loss, and Life-Threatening Illness* (Champaign, IL: Research Press, 1993).

2. J. A. Sanford, *Between People: Communicating One-to-One* (Ramsey, NJ: Paulist Press, 1982), 28.

3. H. J. Clinebell Jr., *Basic Types of Pastoral Counseling* (Nashville: Abington, 1966).

4. J. Stairs, *Listening for the Soul: Pastoral Care and Spiritual Direction* (Minneapolis: Fortress, 2000).

5. Egan, *Exercises in Helping Skills*; Hill and O'Brien, eds., *Helping Skills*; Hammond, et. al., *Improving Therapeutic Communication*; Larson, *The Helper's Journey*.

6. R. Dilts, *Applications of Neuro-Linguistic Programming* (Cupertino, CA: Meta, 1983).

7. R. S. Hebert, M. W. Jenkes, D. E. Ford, D. R. O'Connor, and L. A. Cooper, "Patient Perspectives on Spirituality and the Patient-Physician Relationship," *Journal of General Internal Medicine* 16 (2001): 685–92; E. J. Taylor, "Client Perspectives about Nurse Requisites for Spiritual Caregiving," *Applied Nursing Research* (2007): 44–46.

8. Carkhuff, *The Art of Helping*; Hill and O'Brien, eds., *Helping Skills*.

9. J. O'Connor and J. Seymour, *Introducing Neuro-Linguistic Programming: Psychological Skills for Understanding and Influencing People* (London: Thorsons, 1995).

10. Hill and O'Brien, eds., *Helping Skills*.

11. Ibid.

12. Ibid.

13. Ibid.; Goodman and Esterly, *The Talk Book*; Larson, *The Helper's Journey*.

14. Hill and O'Brien, eds., *Helping Skills*.

15. K. Fischer, "Working with the Emotions in Spiritual Direction: Seven Guiding Principles," *Presence: An International Journal of Spiritual Direction,* 12, no. 3 (2006): 26–35.

16. Larson, *The Helper's Journey*.

17. Hammond, Hepworth, and Smith, *Improving Therapeutic Communication*; C. B. Traux and R. R. Carkhuff, *Toward Effective Counseling and Psychotherapy: Training and Practice* (Chicago: Aldine, 1967); Goodman and Esterly, *The Talk Book*.

18. Hill and O'Brien, eds., *Helping Skills*, 122.

19. Carkhuff, *The Art of Helping*; Egan, *Exercises in Helping Skills*; Hill and O'Brien, eds., *Helping Skills*; Goodman and Esterly, *The Talk Book*; Larson, *The Helper's Journey*; Hammond and Hepworth and Smith, *Improving therapeutic communication*; Hill and O'Brien, eds., *Helping Skills*; G. Egan, *The Skilled Helper: A Problem-Management and Opportunity-Development Approach to Helping*, 7th ed. (Pacific Grove, CA: Brooks/Cole, 2002).

20. Egan, *The Skilled Helper*.

21. Hill and O'Brien, eds., *Helping Skills*; Hammond, Hepworth, and Smith, *Improving Therapeutic Communication*.

22. Egan, *Exercises in Helping Skills*; Hammond, Helpworth, and Smith, *Improving Therapeutic Communication*.

23. Egan, *The Skilled Helper*; Hammond, Hepworth, and Smith, *Improving Therapeutic Communication*.

24. R. R. Carkhuff, *Helping and Human Relations: A Primer for Lay and Professional Helpers, vol. 1: Selection and Training* (New York: Holt, Rinehart, & Winston, 1969).

25. Hammond, Helpworth, and Smith, *Improving Therapeutic Communication*.

26. Carkhuff, *Helping and Human Relations*.

27. R. J. Lovinger, "Religious Issues," in *The Counseling Sourcebook: A Practical Reference on Contemporary Issues,* ed. J. L. Ronch, W. Van Ornum, and N. C. Stilwell (New York: Crossroad, 1994), 202–22; E. J. Taylor, *Spiritual Care: Nursing Research, Theory, and Practice* (Upper Saddle River, NJ: Prentice Hall, 2002); R. J. Lovinger, *Religion and Counseling: The Psychological Impact of Religious Belief* (New York: Continuum, 1990); Hill and O'Brien, eds., *Helping Skills*.

28. Hill and O'Brien, eds., *Helping Skills*.

Chapter 6: Verbal Responses to Spiritual Distress: Macro-skills

1. J. L. Griffith and M. E. Griffith, *Encountering the Sacred in Psychotherapy* (New York: Guilford, 2002).

2. F. Gibson, *The Past in the Present: Using Reminiscence in the Health and Social Care* (Baltimore: Health Professions Press, 2004); E. J. Taylor, "The Story behind the Story: The Use of Storytelling in Spiritual Caregiving," *Seminars in Oncology Nursing* 13, no. 4 (1997): 252–54.

3. H. J. M. Nouwen, *Reaching Out* (Garden City, NJ: Doubleday, 1975).

4. H. Brody, *Stories of Sickness* (New Haven: Yale University, 1987); J. S. Savage, *Listening and Caring Skills in Ministry: A Guide for Pastors, Counselors, and Small Groups* (Nashville: Abington, 1996); J. Kane, *How to Heal: A Guide for Caregivers.* (New York: Allworth Press, 2003); Taylor, *The Story Behind the Story.*

5. Kane, *How to Heal.*

6. E. Hinterkopf, *Integrating Spirituality in Counseling: A Manual for Using the Experiential Focusing Method* (Alexandria, VA: American Counseling Association, 1998); E. T. Gendlin, *Focusing*, 2nd ed. (New York: Bantam, 1981).

7. Ibid.

8. Ibid.

9. Griffith and Griffith, *Encountering the Sacred in Psychotherapy.*

10. J. E. Bower, B. E. Meyerowitz, K. A. Desmond, C. A. Bernaards, J. H. Rowland, and P. A. Ganz, "Perceptions of Positive Meaning and Vulnerability following Breast Cancer: Predictors and Outcomes among Long-Term Breast Cancer Survivors," *Annals of Behavioral Medicine* 29 (2005): 236–45; S. C. Sodergren, M. E. Hyland, A. Crawford, and M. R. Partridge, "Positivity in Illness: Self-delusion or Existential Growth?" *British Journal of Health Psychology* 9 (2004): 163–74; J. A. Updegraff and S. E. Taylor, "From Vulnerability to Growth: Positive and Negative Effects of Stressful Life Events," in *Loss and Trauma: General and Close Relationship Perspectives*, ed. J. H. Harvey and E. D. Miller (Philadelphia: Brunner-Routledge, 2000), 3–28; J. Violanti, D. Paton, and C. Dun-

ning, eds., *Posttraumatic Stress Interventions* (Springfield, IL: Charles C. Thomas, 2000).

11. D. G. Cruess, M. H. Antoni, B. A. McGregor, K. M. Kilbourn, A. E. Boyers, S. M. Alferi, et al., "Cognitive-Behavioral Stress Management Reduces Serum Cortisol by Enhancing Benefit Finding among Women Being Treated for Early Stage Breast Cancer," *Psychosomatic Medicine* 62 (2000): 304–8.

12. S. Grossman, A. A. Wyszynski, L. Barkin, and V. Schwartz, "When Patients Ask about the Spiritual: A Primer," in *Manual of Psychiatric Care for the Medically Ill*, ed. A. A. Wyszynski and B. Wyszynski (Washington, DC: American Psychiatric Publishing, 2005), 237–43.

13. Violanti, Paton, and Dunning, eds., *Posttraumatic Stress Interventions*.

14. Griffith and Griffith, *Encountering the Sacred in Psychotherapy*.

15. Ibid.

16. E. C. Kennedy and S. Charles, *On Becoming a Counselor: A Basic Guide for Non-Professional Counselors* (New York: Continuum, 1990); K. Shea, "Reframing: A Fresh Outlook Helps Patients Envision Positive Outcomes," *NurseWeek*, November 1, 2004.

17. D. P. Barkwell, "Ascribed Meaning: A Critical Factor in Coping and Pain Attenuation in Patients with Cancer-Related Pain," *Journal of Palliative Care* 7, no. 3 (1991): 5–14.

18. Shea, "Reframing: A Fresh Outlook Helps Patients Envision Positive Outcomes"; J. O'Connor and J. Seymour, *Introducing Neuro-Linguistic Programming: Psychological Skills for Understanding and Influencing People* (London: Thorsons, 1995).

19. R. J. Lovinger, "Religious Issues," in *The Counseling Sourcebook: A Practical Reference on Contemporary Issues*, ed. J. L. Ronch, W. Van Ornum, and N. C. Stilwell (New York: Crossroad, 1994), 202–22.

20. J. S. Levin, *God, Faith and Health: Exploring the Spirituality-Healing Connection* (New York: John Wiley, 2001) ; C. M. Puchalski, R. E. Dorff, and I. Y. Hendi, "Spirituality, Religion, and Healing in Palliative Care," *Clinical Geriatric Medicine* 20 (2004): 689–714.

21. G. R. Winslow and B. W. Winslow, "Examining the Ethics of Praying with Patients," *Holistic Nursing Practice* 17, no. 4 (2003): 170–77.

22. M. Buber, cited in H. J. Clinebell Jr., *Basic Types of Pastoral Counseling* (Nashville: Abington, 1966), 261.

23. G. H. Gallup Jr., *Religion in America* (Princeton, NJ: Princeton Religion Research Center, 1996); J. A. McNeill, "Assessing Clinical Outcomes: Patient Satisfaction with Pain Management," *Journal of Pain and Symptom Management* 16 (1998): 29–40;

24. E. J. Taylor, "Prayer's Clinical Issues and Implications," *Holistic Nursing Practice* 17 (2003): 179–88; R. J. Lovinger, *Religion and Counseling: The Psychological Impact of Religious Belief* (New York: Continuum, 1990); Clinebell, *Basic Types of Pastoral Counseling*; Lovinger, *Religion and Counseling*.

Chapter 7: FAQs

1. C. E. Hill and K. M. O'Brien, eds., *Helping Skills: Facilitating Exploration, Insight, and Action* (Washington, DC: American Psychological Association, 1999).

2. Ibid.

3. M. F. Highfield, "Spiritual Health of Oncology Patients: Nurse and Patient Perspectives," *Cancer Nursing* 15 (1992): 1–8; P. G. Reed, "Preferences for Spiritually Related Nursing Interventions among Terminally Ill and Nonterminally Ill Hospitalized Adults and Well Adults," *Applied Nursing Research* 4 (1991): 122–28.

4. E. J. Taylor, "Client Perspectives about Nurse Requisites for Spiritual Caregiving," *Applied Nursing Research* (2007): 44–46.

5. E. J. Taylor, *Spiritual Care: Nursing Research, Theory, and Practice* (Upper Saddle River, NJ: Prentice Hall, 2002).

6. R. G. Tedeschi and L. G. Calhoun, *Trauma and Transformation: Growing in the Aftermath of Suffering* (Thousand Oaks, CA: Sage, 1995); J. A. Updegraff and S. E. Taylor, "From Vulnerability to Growth: Positive and Negative Effects of Stressful Life Events," in *Loss and Trauma: General and Close Relationship Perspectives*, ed. J. H. Harvey and E D. Miller (Philadelphia: Brunner-Routledge, 2000), 3–28; J. Violanti, D. Paton, and C. Dunning, eds., *Posttraumatic Stress Interventions* (Springfield, IL: Charles C. Thomas, 2000).

7. J. S. Carpenter, D. Y. Brockopp, and M. A. Andrykowski, "Self-Transformation as a Factor in the Self-Esteem and Well-Being of Breast Cancer Survivors," *Journal of Advanced Nursing* 29 (1999): 1402–11; E. J. Taylor, "Transformation of Tragedy among Women Surviving Breast Cancer," *Oncology Nursing Forum* 27 (2000): 781–88.

8. K. I. Pargament, H. G. Koenig, and L. M. Perez, "The Many Methods of Religious Coping: Development and Initial Testing of the RCOPE," *Journal of Clinical Psychology* 56 (2000): 519–43; K. I. Pargament, B. J. Zinnbauer, A. B. Scott, E. M. Butter, J. Zerowin, and P. Stanik, "Red Flags and Religious Coping: Identifying Some Religious Warning Signs among People in Crisis," *Journal of Clinical Psychology* 54 (1998): 77–89; H. G. Koenig, K. I. Pargament, and J. Nielsen, "Religious Coping and Health Status in Medically Ill Hospitalized Older Adults," *Journal of Nervous and Mental Disease* 186 (1998): 513–21; J. R. Mickley, K. I. Pargament, C. R. Brant, and K. M. Hipp, "God and the Search for Meaning among Hospice Caregivers," *Hospice Journal* 13, no. 4 (1998): 1–17.

9. R. J. Lovinger, *Religion and Counseling: The Psychological Impact of Religious Belief* (New York: Continuum, 1990), 33.

10. R. B. Connors Jr. and M. L. Smith, "Religious Insistence on Medical Treatment: Christian Theology and Re-Imagination," *Hastings Center Report* 26, no. 4 (1996): 23–30.

11. J. A. Sanford, *Between People: Communicating One-to-One* (Ramsey, NJ: Paulist Press, 1982), 71.

12. S. Grossman, A. A. Wyszynski, L. Barkin, and V. Schwartz, "When Patients Ask about the Spiritual: A Primer," in *Manual of Psychiatric Care for the Medically Ill*, ed. A. A. Wyszynski and B. Wyszynski (Washington, DC: American Psychiatric Publishing, 2005), 237–43.

13. Lovinger, *Religion and Counseling*, 139.

14. K. L. Mauk and N. K. Schmidt, *Spiritual Care in Nursing Practice* (Philadelphia: Lippincott Williams & Wilkins, 2004); L. E. Sullivan, ed., *Healing and Restoring: Health and Medicine in the World's Religious Traditions* (New York: Macmillan, 1989); R. L. Numbers and D. W. Amundsen, *Caring and Curing: Health and Medicine in the Western Religious Traditions* (New York: Macmillan, 1986); Taylor, *Spiritual Care*.

15. Taylor, *Spiritual Care*; K. Massey, G. Fitchett, and P. A. Roberts, "Assessment and Diagnosis in Spiritual Care," in *Spiritual Care in Nursing Practice*, ed. K. L. Mauk and N. K. Schmidt (Philadelphia: Lippincott Williams & Wilkins, 2004), 209–42.

16. Grossman, Wyszynski, Barkin, and Schwartz, "When Patients Ask about the Spiritual: A Primer"; Taylor, *Spiritual Care*; B. M. Dossey, "Holistic Modalities and Healing Moments," *American Journal of Nursing* 98 (1998): 44–47; J. R. Dudley, C. Smith, and M. B. Millison, "Unfinished Business: Assessing the Spiritual Needs of Hospice Clients," *American Journal of Hospice and Palliative Care* 12, no. 2 (1995): 30–37; C. M. Puchalski, "Spirituality and End of Life Care: A Time for Listening and Caring," *Journal of Palliative Medicine* 5 (2002): 289–94.

17. J. L. Griffith and M. E. Griffith, *Encountering the Sacred in Psychotherapy* (New York: Guilford, 2002), 273–74.

18. Grossman, Wyszynski, Barkin, and Schwartz, "When Patients Ask about the Spiritual: A Primer."

19. L. Aveling, S. Sorajjakool, and R. Pulliam, "Working with Difficult Patients: Spiritual Care Approaches," In *Spirituality, Health, and Wholeness: An Introductory Guide for Health Care Professionals*, ed. S. Sirajjakool & H. Lamberton (New York: Haworth Press, 2004), 161–74.

20. Ibid.

21. W. Wordsworth, "Ode: Initiations of Immortality, from Recollections of Early Childhood," cited in B. W. Talbert, "Partners with Listening Hearts: Some Thoughts on Christian Formation in Families," *Journal of Family Ministry* 14, no. 1 (2000): 20–29.